CLASSROOM PIVOTAL RESPONSE TEACHING FOR CHILDREN WITH AUTISM

Classroom Pivotal Response Teaching
for Children with Autism

Aubyn C. Stahmer
Jessica Suhrheinrich
Sarah Reed
Laura Schreibman
Cynthia Bolduc

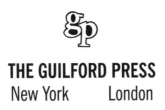

THE GUILFORD PRESS
New York   London

Printed in the United States of America

This book is printed on acid-free paper.

Last digit is print number: 9 8 7 6 5 4 3 2 1

The authors have checked with sources believed to be reliable in their efforts to provide information that is complete and generally in accord with the standards of practice that are accepted at the time of publication. However, in view of the possibility of human error or changes in behavioral, mental health, or medical sciences, neither the authors, nor the editor and publisher, nor any other party who has been involved in the preparation or publication of this work warrants that the information contained herein is in every respect accurate or complete, and they are not responsible for any errors or omissions or the results obtained from the use of such information. Readers are encouraged to confirm the information contained in this book with other sources.

Library of Congress Cataloging-in-Publication Data

Classroom pivotal response teaching for children with autism / Aubyn C. Stahmer ... [et al.].
    p. cm.
    Summary: "Classroom Pivotal Response Teaching, or CPRT, was developed to help meet the educational needs of young children with autism. CPRT (originally called Pivotal Response Training or Treatment) is a form of naturalistic behavioral intervention, based on the principles of applied behavior analysis (ABA), and is soundly supported in the scientific literature. This manual will describe the components of CPRT and how to implement the approach in your classroom. Although this manual is geared primarily toward preschool through grade 3 teachers, CPRT strategies can be used by a variety of professionals. Speech and language pathologists, occupational therapists, behavior specialists, psychologists, and other teaching professionals may all find CPRT a valuable strategy. Additionally, the techniques in this manual may be useful with typically developing children and those with a variety of special needs. Most children can benefit from this structured, systematic approach that utilizes naturally occurring teaching opportunities. One of the strengths of this approach is that it is adaptable to a wide range of teaching goals and service settings. All who teach are encouraged to integrate CPRT into their existing strategies as often as possible"—Provided by publisher.
    Includes bibliographical references and index.
    ISBN 978-1-60918-241-0 (pbk.)
    1. Autistic children—Education. 2. Autistic children—Behavior modification. I. Stahmer, Aubyn C. II. Title.
    LC4717.C53 2011+
    371.94—dc22
                                   2010051672

About the Authors

Aubyn C. Stahmer, PhD, is Research Scientist at the Child and Adolescent Services Research Center (CASRC); Associate Project Scientist in the Department of Psychology at the University of California, San Diego (UCSD); and Research Director at Rady Children's Hospital Autism Discovery Institute. She has over 20 years of experience in working with children with autism and using Pivotal Response Training (PRT). A major goal of her research has been to examine educational services for young children with autism in order to inform the translation of evidence-based practice into community settings. Dr. Stahmer has extensive experience with training teachers in behavioral and developmental techniques, and with developing clinically relevant ongoing program fidelity-of-implementation procedures.

Jessica Suhrheinrich, PhD, is a postdoctoral researcher at UCSD and CASRC. She is an experienced PRT trainer. Her primary area of research interest involves examining the use of PRT by classroom teachers and the best methods of training teachers to use PRT in the classroom. Before beginning graduate school, Dr. Suhrheinrich was a classroom teacher herself, and thus she has an excellent understanding of the barriers to implementing evidence-based practice in community settings.

Sarah Reed, MA, is a doctoral student in the UCSD Autism Intervention Research Program. Her graduate research focuses on the implementation of evidence-based treatments in community environments and on optimal ways to translate intervention research across service delivery settings. Her primary research interest involves continuing to examine the effectiveness of PRT with groups of students, as this is the service reality for many settings. Clinically, Ms. Reed has extensive experience in implementing naturalistic behavioral interventions with children with autism, as well as in providing training to parents, clinicians, and students in these methods.

Laura Schreibman, PhD, is Distinguished Professor of Psychology at UCSD. For the past 40 years, she has conducted research examining intervention methods for children with autism. She is one of the developers of PRT, and is an author of numerous peer-reviewed publications examining the efficacy of this intervention. Dr. Schreibman is also the author of three books on autism, the most recent of which is *The Science and Fiction of Autism*. She has experience in the development of behavioral assessment measures of fidelity of implementation, as well as in treatment adaptation.

Cynthia Bolduc, MA, has been teaching children in special education for 10 years and specifically serving children with autism for 7 years. She is trained in several evidence-based techniques used with this population, including PRT. Ms. Bolduc uses PRT in her program as part of an eclectic set of interventions. She has completed a master's degree with an emphasis in educating children with autism.

About the CPRT Advisory Board

Patricia Belden, MA, has recently retired after devoting most of her 35 years in education to working with children with autism and their families within the public school setting. She has served in the capacities of teacher, school principal, and districtwide administrator. In her effort to support preservice teachers, she has been a master teacher and a student teacher supervisor for San Diego State University (SDSU) in conjunction with the SDSU autism specialization master's degree program. Ms. Belden is currently a part-time faculty member at the University of San Diego in the special education credentialing and master's degree programs.

Thesa Jolly, MEd, has recently retired after working in the field of special education for over 35 years. She has worked with infants and preschool children with special needs in home- and center-based programs in the United States as well as overseas. She has been a mentor teacher and master teacher with the San Diego Unified School District. Ms. Jolly's focus has been on incorporating PRT techniques into a developmental curriculum that can benefit all children in her classroom.

Catherine Pope, MA, has been working with preschool students with autism for the past 10 years. She received her teaching credential and master's degree in education with a specialization in autism from SDSU. She incorporates research-based practices into her classroom curriculum, which includes principles of applied behavior analysis. Ms. Pope has implemented paraprofessional training in PRT in the classroom, and she is a coauthor of a publication on training paraprofessionals to use behavioral strategies.

Linda Reeve, MA, NBCT, holds a teaching credential and a master's degree in early childhood special education. She has been working with children on the autism spectrum in public schools as a classroom teacher and early childhood autism specialist since 1992. Ms. Reeve consults with districts throughout San Diego County on developing public school programs for their students with autism. She brings experience in developing and supervising behavioral programs in home and school settings. She also supervises university students in their teacher training programs and sits on several autism advisory boards.

Lauren Ungar, MEd, has been in the field of education for 6 years. She is currently teaching elementary students with severe needs in kindergarten to third grade. PRT is among the many methodological approaches Ms. Ungar uses within her classroom to help serve students with autism and other diagnoses.

Acknowledgments

This Classroom Pivotal Response Teaching (CPRT) manual is a result of ongoing collaboration among researchers, classroom teachers, and program administrators. In addition to the many children who have taught us about the challenges and joys of teaching students with autism, we especially want to thank the following individuals for their contributions to the development of this manual:

- The Institute of Education Sciences at the U.S. Department of Education (Grant No. R324B070027) for providing funding both for the development of this manual and for several of the research studies informing the project.

- *Drs. Robert and Lynn Koegel*, who, together with Laura Schreibman, conducted the original Pivotal Response Training (PRT) research and developed PRT as a manualized intervention. Your dedication to improving the lives of children with autism and their families has inspired us to conduct this community-based work. In addition, we are grateful to the many researchers who have carefully examined the use of PRT in home, community, and classroom environments, and to the parents and teachers who have learned to use these strategies in the real world.

- Our partners on the CPRT Advisory Board—*Patricia Belden, Thesa Jolly, Catherine Pope, Linda Reeve*, and *Lauren Ungar*—for dedicating so much time over the past few years to helping us develop the CPRT manual. Thank you for sharing your teaching wisdom; providing such detailed and valuable input on our many, many drafts of these materials; sharing your materials and examples of how you adapted the procedures for your unique students and classrooms; and keeping us grounded in the real world.

- *Lauren Brookman-Frazee, Laura Hall,* and *Lauren Loos* for sharing your clinical and research expertise in autism, and helping us integrate our own knowledge and translate the intervention strategies in a user-friendly and practical manner.

- All those who reviewed earlier drafts and helped to shape the final manual: *Genevieve Bolduc, Michelle Carney, Mary Lou Evans, Josh Feder, Georgeanne Gedney, Rebecca Gutierrez, Kay Holman, Zinnia Piotrowski,* and *Lisa Ruble.* We would also like to thank *Caitlin Loos* at *Caitlin.e.loos Marketing and Graphic Design* for providing the original layout and design, and *Glenda Rogers* for developing the CPRT logo.

Contents

How to Use This Manual

What Is CPRT and Who Should Use This Approach?

Classroom Pivotal Response Teaching (CPRT), was developed to help meet the educational needs of young children with autism. CPRT, originally called **Pivotal Response Training or Treatment (PRT)**, is a form of naturalistic behavioral intervention based on the principles of **Applied Behavior Analysis (ABA)**, and is soundly supported in the scientific literature. This manual describes the components of CPRT and discusses how to implement the approach in your classroom.

Although this manual is geared primarily toward preschool through grade 3 teachers, CPRT strategies can be used by a variety of professionals. Speech and language pathologists, occupational therapists, behavior specialists, psychologists, and other teaching professionals may all find CPRT a valuable strategy. Additionally, the techniques in this manual may be useful with typically developing children and those with a variety of special needs. Most children can benefit from this structured, systematic approach that utilizes naturally occurring teaching opportunities. One of the strengths of this approach is that it is adaptable to a wide range of teaching goals and service settings. All who teach are encouraged to integrate CPRT into their existing strategies as often as possible.

CPRT is for:

- *Teachers and school staff*
- *Students in preschool through grade 3*
- *Special education, general education, and resource settings*

Features of the Manual

Organization of the Manual

We recommend reading this manual from start to finish for optimal comprehension and learning. This does not mean, however, that the entire manual must be read in a single sitting! Different portions of the manual may be useful at different times, depending on your goals for incorporating CPRT into your classroom and your familiarity with this or similar approaches. It is advisable to learn the basics of CPRT and practice the approach with individual students before moving to the more advanced steps of integrating it as a classroomwide approach. To facilitate use of the manual, we have divided it into four parts. Each part has a specific purpose:

- *Part I* introduces the principles of CPRT and explains how to use the intervention with individual students. It is important to be familiar with all the material in *Part I* before moving forward with CPRT.
- *Part II* is designed to teach CPRT implementation with groups of students and classroom adaptation, and it includes many tips and tools to aid this process.
- *Part III* contains information on teaching classroom staff and parents about CPRT, as well as a description of the research support behind the approach that may be useful as you explain your choice of CPRT for your students.
- *Part IV* provides materials such as data collection sheets, summary handouts, and goal development forms to help you use CPRT successfully in your classroom.

Our hope is that you will keep this manual handy even after familiarizing yourself with CPRT and will refer to it as a resource for ideas, troubleshooting, and training materials.

The goal of the following description is to provide a brief overview of the contents of this manual, so you can quickly locate relevant sections and easily find specific information. Particularly as you move from *Part I* to *Part II*, the skills taught in each chapter provide a foundation for the skills following. It can be helpful to think of these skills as a pyramid: The successively higher levels require the levels below them as a base in order to be used effectively. *Figure 1* shows the pyramid of the *CPRT Knowledge Hierarchy*, beginning with the base of understanding ABA and the principles of CPRT. Once you understand these, you can begin to practice implementing them with individual students, and then during group instruction. Next you can start to target specific **Individualized Education Program (IEP)** and curriculum goals using CPRT, integrate the strategies into your classroom, and finally train others to use the techniques.

Part I: Getting Started with CPRT

- *Chapter 1* contains a general introduction to the original PRT protocol, describes the features of autism, and provides information about the main components of CPRT. This chapter also discusses why CPRT may be a good strategy for use in the classroom, what skills can be taught using CPRT, what activities and materials can be used in CPRT, when to use CPRT, and when it may be best to employ another approach.

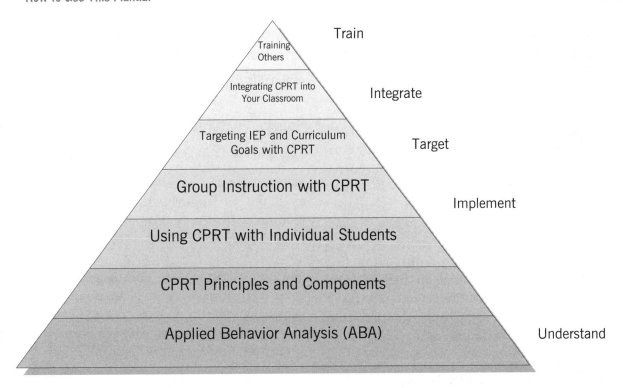

FIGURE 1. **CPRT Knowledge Hierarchy.** This pyramid illustrates how the skills necessary to implement and use PRT in your classroom build upon each other. It is necessary to have a strong foundation in the lower levels of understanding ABA and CPRT components before moving up the pyramid to targeting IEP goals and training others.

- *Chapter 2* contains an overview of ABA, to provide the theoretical background of the CPRT approach. CPRT is based on the principles of ABA, and it is important to understand the patterns of antecedents, behaviors, and consequences before implementing the specific components. In our experience, people who are familiar with ABA are more successful in using CPRT because knowledge of the underlying principles allows them to adapt their skills to their students' needs.

- *Chapter 3* presents the main description of CPRT and explains how to implement the basic components. Each component is followed by good and poor examples of implementation, to clarify the basics of how CPRT works. This chapter will be a valuable reference as you develop your skills in each component of the approach.

Part II: Next Steps with CPRT

- *Chapter 4* covers how to use CPRT with a group of students. Since there can be many teaching settings even within a single classroom (one-on-one teaching, small-group tasks, large-group activities, etc.), this chapter describes how CPRT strategies can be effectively utilized both to address a single student's goals within a group and to conduct maximally effective group instruction.

- *Chapter 5* explains how to use CPRT to meet your students' IEP and curriculum-based goals. The chapter emphasizes addressing a variety of goals in a naturalistic way and explains how to apply CPRT specifically to communication, play, social, and academic goals. Examples of goals are provided for a variety of functioning levels. Each section includes a discussion of where to begin, optimal opportunities to address specific skills, and ways to progress toward meeting your students' goals.

- *Chapter 6* is designed to help you incorporate CPRT into your classroom. This chapter contains information on how to integrate CPRT with your current curricula and standards, utilize CPRT alongside other complementary interventions, identify materials that motivate your students, collect data during CPRT, and target generalization of skills from the start. Several data collection methods are described; choose those that best meet your specific needs. Troubleshooting tips are provided at the end of this chapter.

Part III: Resources and Support

- *Chapter 7* contains information and materials for training your classroom staff both effectively and efficiently. Teaching students with autism is the collaborative work of a dedicated team, and sharing CPRT with all professionals who work with your students will facilitate student learning and progress.

- *Chapter 8* helps you explain CPRT to parents, with the hope that they will also use these naturalistic strategies at home. Involving parents is likely to promote better generalization and maintenance of skills.

- *Chapter 9* details the research supporting the effectiveness of CPRT in teaching students with autism. This chapter can be used to support your choice of CPRT as an effective and evidence-based strategy when you are discussing your teaching methods with others.

Part IV: Reproducible Handouts

Part IV contains all the blank forms and other materials discussed earlier in the manual.

Special Features

Examples of Completed Forms

Throughout the text, you will see several examples of completed forms related to planning, student goals, and data collection. All the forms used in these examples are available in *Part IV* of the manual, and you are encouraged to photocopy and utilize these forms when implementing CPRT in your classroom. Copies of the forms are also available to print directly from the DVD accompanying this manual.

Glossary

A *Glossary* of behavioral terms and related vocabulary is provided at the end of the book. Words that appear in **boldface** throughout the text are further defined in the *Glossary*.

Suggested Readings

A list of *Suggested Readings* is also provided at the end of the book. This is by no means an exhaustive bibliography; it is intended simply as a guide to the research in this field.

Training Lectures

The DVD accompanying this manual contains two sets of CPRT training lectures, to assist teachers in understanding CPRT and to help train support staff. These presentations cover several topics in the book. Teachers and support staff can watch the narrated, animated lectures as part of training. Illustrative videos are included in the presentations.

Icons

Throughout the manual, you will see several icons highlighting important points and features of the text. These icons are intended to facilitate reading and provide quick tips. The specific meanings of the icons are listed below.

 Resources: The book icon indicates that additional resources pertaining to this area are available in the manual. For example, this icon appears next to the discussion on CPRT and data collection, because a variety of data collection worksheets are included in *Part IV*.

 Activities and Materials: The toy icon highlights suggestions for specific teaching materials or activities that are well suited for CPRT. One of the strengths of CPRT is the absence of specific, necessary materials, which makes it inexpensive and portable. However, the absence of specified materials also occasionally requires creativity, and these items are intended to inspire new ideas and help you to use CPRT in a wide variety of situations.

 Notes and Forms: The notepad icon indicates an opportunity to take notes related to a specific topic or to fill out a particular worksheet included in *Part IV*. These opportunities are intended to facilitate active reading of the manual and to help you relate the content to the reality of your classroom as you read.

 Troubleshooting: The tool icon is a sign for troubleshooting tips and tricks to resolve issues that may arise in utilizing CPRT. These sections address common problems seen with implementation, student response, and staff training. There is also a more extensive list of troubleshooting tips at the end of *Chapter 6*.

 Information: The "i" icon directs you to further information on a particular subject. These points are intended as a guide to outside resources relevant to CPRT and teaching students with autism.

PART I

Getting Started with CPRT

CHAPTER 1
Introduction to CPRT

CHAPTER OVERVIEW

Classroom Pivotal Response Teaching (CPRT) was developed to help meet the educational needs of students with autism. Autism is a pervasive developmental disorder characterized by impairments in communication and social interaction, as well as restricted and repetitive interests and behaviors. The purpose of developing CPRT was to adapt the research-supported components of Pivotal Response Training (PRT) to the demands of teaching within a classroom environment. CPRT is fun to use, versatile, and adaptable, and its effectiveness is acknowledged by teachers who use it and by research. The components of CPRT are designed to be used throughout the day in a variety of settings, with materials and activities you commonly use in the classroom. CPRT can be used to teach communication, play, social, and academic skills, and it promotes generalization of skills.

The following sections are included:

What Is Autism?

How CPRT Is Used to Teach Children with Autism

Why Should I Use CPRT in My Classroom?

What Skills Can I Teach Using CPRT?

What Activities or Materials Can Be Used in CPRT?

When Should I Use CPRT?

When CPRT Isn't the Best Choice

Classroom Pivotal Response Teaching (CPRT) is a naturalistic behavioral intervention that is soundly supported in the scientific literature and has been developed for use during day-to-day classroom activities. The intervention focuses on student motivation and involves presenting clear opportunities to respond, supporting student skill use, and providing appropriate consequences based on student behavior. CPRT can be used to teach a variety of skills, including communication, play, peer social interaction, self-initiations, academic skills, and joint attention.

As rates of autism increase, there is growing pressure on teachers to provide high-quality specialized programming. Managing the highly varied needs of students with autism can be a challenge, and undoubtedly many factors go into deciding which strategies to use with these students. Teachers report using a particular intervention because it "makes sense," or because they try it and find that it works.

Our hope is that you will choose to implement CPRT in your classroom, based on the intuitive nature of the approach as well as the solid research base.

Teachers we have worked with find CPRT to be fun and easy to implement with their students. When learning CPRT, teachers often report that they are already using many of the components without having an explicit name for their techniques. Learning CPRT is not likely to require a dramatic change in the way you interact with your students; instead, it provides a way to label and enhance your teaching methods so that you can maximize student achievement, easily identify your strengths and weaknesses, and train others to use the same approach. CPRT was designed specifically for use in the classroom; this manual includes the necessary tools and resources to make CPRT a comprehensive teaching strategy rather than just an intervention.

What Is Autism?

Within the last 20 years, estimates of the number of children with an educational categorization of autism have increased to about 1 in 100. This dramatic increase has influenced the quality and type of educational opportunities available for children with autism.

Research shows that early intervention and educational services can greatly improve outcomes for some students with autism. These findings have led to more demand for effective, usable programs that meet the needs of classroom staff and their students.

Autism is a pervasive developmental disorder, meaning that students with autism have problems in all areas of development. Students with autism face challenges with communication and social skills, and can show restricted, repetitive, and stereotyped patterns of behavior. Some students with autism do not develop speech. Students who do learn to talk often develop unusual speech patterns (e.g., monotone inflection) or have difficulty using language on their own. In addition, the development and use of gestures such as pointing is often impaired, furthering overall communication problems. Social deficits may include avoidance of eye contact, difficulty interacting with classmates, and odd or inappropriate play. Severe repetitive behavior can also interfere with learning. The severity of these symptoms varies across students, and behaviors and skills will change over time with intervention and development. Students with autism are likely to have some difficulty with almost every aspect of social and psychological development.

Up to 50% of children with autism have impaired cognitive development and will score in the moderately to severely delayed range on standardized assessments. Although some students with autism can have average or even above-average ability in some areas, they may still experience difficulty with academics and almost always have a hard time socially. A student with autism may be able to recite the dialogue from a movie, complete with voices and expression, yet may not vary his voice when speaking with others. He may have no interest in playing with classmates, instead choosing to memorize a map of the United States or spin the wheels of a car he has turned upside down. Another student may want to play with friends but doesn't know how to join in a group activity. As she gets older, she may seek attention from other people, but only to talk about her own interests. A young student with autism may show a remarkable ability to identify letters and numbers and "read" words, but may still have delayed language. An older student with autism may be able to do well on standardized academic tests, and may yet have difficulty making it through school without special accommodations. One of the most notable features of autism is the variability in cognitive and communication abilities among those diagnosed with it.

Autism is commonly seen as a spectrum of disorders. The current spectrum includes:

- Autistic Disorder: the diagnosis given to students with "classic" symptoms of autism.
- Asperger's Disorder: a diagnosis used for students with average to above-average cognitive abilities and less severe communication problems.
- Pervasive Developmental Disorder Not Otherwise Specified (PDD-NOS): a "catch-all" category used for students who have many symptoms associated with Autistic Disorder but do not meet the full diagnostic criteria.

In your classroom, you are likely to have students who fit into all of these specific diagnoses identified under the educational category of autism. Because autism is a spectrum of disorders, each student will be different and will require an individualized program of services.

References for the information discussed in each chapter can be found in the *Suggested Readings* list at the end of the book. A review of the research supporting PRT is provided in *Chapter 9*. Both of these provide more information about the scientific basis of the topics discussed in this manual.

For more information about the characteristics of autism, we recommend *www.autismspeaks.org* and *www.autism-society.org*.

How CPRT Is Used to Teach Children with Autism

CPRT has been adapted for classroom use from a program called **Pivotal Response Training (PRT)**. PRT is based on a series of studies identifying important treatment components (again, see *Chapter 9* for a complete description of the scientific support for PRT). The "pivotal" responses trained in PRT are motivation, initiation, and responsivity to multiple cues (i.e., increasing breadth of attention). Each interaction with a student involves a teacher's providing a cue or opportunity to respond, the student's exhibiting a behavior, and the teacher's providing feedback to the student. Specific components for presenting a cue include gaining the student's attention; providing a clear and developmentally appropriate instruction; and using shared control of tasks and activities, including providing the child a choice of activity or materials, and taking turns. Cues in a teaching activity include providing a mixture of easy and difficult tasks and giving the student an opportunity to respond to multiple cues if appropriate. If needed, the teacher can provide specific prompts to help the student make an appropriate response. Once the student responds, the teacher provides reinforcement based on the response, and can reward a goal-directed attempt (a good try); the teacher also makes sure the reward is related to the activity. (See *Figure 1.1* for a list of CPRT components, and *Chapter 3* for a detailed description of each component.) The use of these components leads to increased motivation and learning for many children with autism.

An independent review of the research base recommends PRT as an efficacious, evidence-based intervention for children with autism.

Research highlights the effectiveness of PRT as a teaching tool for skills often targeted in special education programs, such as communication, joint attention, play skills, peer social interaction, and independent work completion. In research comparing

CPRT Components

Cue

Student Attention
Be sure your student is paying attention before you provide a cue.

Clear and Appropriate Instruction
Provide clear and appropriate cues that are at, or just above, your student's developmental level.

Easy and Difficult Tasks (Maintenance/Acquisition)
Provide a mixture of easy and difficult tasks to increase motivation.

Shared Control (Student Choice/Turn Taking)
Share control by following your student's lead, providing choices of activities and materials, and taking turns with your student.

Multiple Cues (Broadening Attention)
Use multiple examples of materials and concepts to ensure broad understanding.

Present opportunities to respond that require your student to attend to multiple aspects of the learning materials.

Student Behavior or Response

Response

Direct Reinforcement
Provide reinforcement that is naturally or directly related to the activity or behavior.

Contingent Consequence (Immediate and Appropriate)
Present consequences immediately, based on the student's response.

Reinforcement of Attempts
Reward good trying to encourage your student to try again in the future.

FIGURE 1.1. CPRT Components. This figure summarizes the components of CPRT and indicates which components are related to cue presentation and teacher response.

PRT to a more structured approach called Discrete Trial Teaching (DTT), children learning via PRT showed greater gains in communication skills, better generalization of skills, and greater reduction in challenging behaviors.

Teachers and researchers have worked together to modify PRT strategies to better fit into a classroom environment. We call this new method Classroom Pivotal Response Teaching or CPRT, to highlight changes that make the program more suited to group classroom environments.

Why Should I Use CPRT in My Classroom?

PRT, the basis for CPRT, is an effective, research-supported intervention that can be easily adopted into your repertoire of teaching strategies. PRT has undergone many years of development, refinement, and effectiveness testing. Several major organizations have determined that PRT is an effective strategy for students with autism, including the National Research Council (2001) and the National Autism Center's (2009) National Standards Project. Additionally, teachers use CPRT and tell us how beneficial it is for their students.

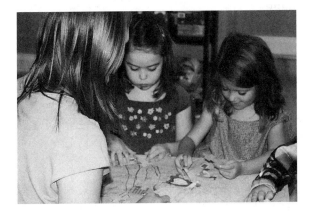

"CPRT differs from other strategies I use with my students, because it allows me to present learning opportunities using the toys and activities that motivate them the most. We all enjoy the fun of playing together."—Preschool special education teacher

- *CPRT is fun!* Students typically enjoy CPRT because a primary focus of the program is increasing their motivation. Students help to select the materials and activities, and as a result are likely to be more engaged in the learning process than when the activity is chosen by a teacher. CPRT is often fun for teachers as well, because students tend to be compliant, motivated, and unlikely to engage in escape/avoidance behavior such as crying. Additionally, because CPRT is a naturalistic intervention, the student–teacher exchange can be conducted in multiple settings and is less structured than in other behavioral strategies. Many teachers enjoy this more natural style of interaction and prefer CPRT to more structured strategies.

- *CPRT is versatile!* It can be used throughout the day, in a variety of settings, and with multiple instructors. There are no specific materials required to use CPRT, so it is also inexpensive and portable. Teachers, classroom staff, and therapists using CPRT with their students incorporate instructional goals into naturally occurring learning opportunities. These strategies can continue to be used as a student rides the bus, participates in after-school activities, and interacts with family members at home. CPRT can be easily integrated into the school day to work on educational goals such as communication, joint attention, social interaction, academic skills, independent work, object play, and general initiations. Once you learn the intervention, you can use CPRT anywhere—and you are likely to find that you do.

- *CPRT is easy to learn!* Research indicates that parents and providers can be trained quickly in the principles of CPRT, leading to immediate use of CPRT and improved overall quality of services.

- *CPRT is adaptable!* There is no specific curriculum associated with CPRT, so it can be used with any standards or curriculum your school is using. The strategies were developed to meet goals based on student needs, rather than to match a specific curriculum. When using CPRT, you will individualize the teaching moments to meet the academic needs of your students. CPRT can complement and be used alongside approaches such as DTT and Structured Teaching, making it easy to integrate into your current programming.

- *And, Most Important, CPRT Is Effective!* These strategies have been shown to help students learn new language, social, play, and academic skills. One of the critical components of learning is a student's ability to use what he has learned in multiple environments, with varied materials, and with different people. This is called **generalization** of skills. CPRT is effective in promoting generalization of skills because teachers help their students learn in a natural way. For example, students can learn to identify colors by jumping on colored dots in gym class, requesting crayons during an art activity, or sharing Skittles at lunch. These activities involve different settings, teachers, and materials, but the instructional goal is the same. Another benefit is that skills learned via CPRT will be reinforced in other situations. When a

student is at the ice cream store, she can request the "brown" ice cream, and her behavior will be reinforced by receiving the flavor she wants. Another aspect of learning is the maintenance of skills. This means that a student remembers what he has learned over time. When you teach using CPRT, you increase the likelihood that your student will maintain the skills he has learned because, again, they were presented in a naturalistic way and are continually supported in his everyday environment. A student who has learned to label colors will have an opportunity to practice this skill daily when telling her mom which t-shirt she wants to wear or requesting a ball at recess.

 Check out *Chapter 9* for a full review of the research supporting CPRT.

What Skills Can I Teach Using CPRT?

Communication, play, social, and academic skills can all be taught using CPRT. This manual provides examples of different ways to teach each of these types of skills. When working with an individual student, start by generating a list of activities that can be utilized to target a specific goal for your student.

For example, a student learning to count to 10 can be taught:

- During snack time by counting the number of crackers he wants.

- During an art activity by counting the number of stickers he wants to put on his paper.

- During a reading exercise by counting the number of animals on the page before turning to the next page.

In each of these scenarios, the student must count in order to get access to something he wants. When you are forming groups, consider skills that are goals for several students in your class and put them together.

For example, several students in your class may be learning to read, but they are currently functioning at different levels:

- Jennifer is learning to identify letters.
- Ibrahim is learning phonics.
- Peter is sight-reading short words.

You can target each of these skills not just during a reading lesson, but also at other naturally occurring opportunities throughout the day. Stop in front of the cafeteria door and ask Jennifer to identify the letter C; when she responds correctly, she can enter the cafeteria. Continue by asking Ibrahim what sound C makes, and have Peter attempt to read a short word beginning with C.

What Activities or Materials Can Be Used in CPRT?

CPRT can be used with any activities or materials that interest your students. Motivating your students through activities or topics they enjoy is a key element of CPRT. Therefore, it is important to identify what your students like (perhaps by using a **preference assessment**) and to use these items to provide positive reinforcement. Students may be naturally motivated for an activity in the classroom, or you can incorporate things they enjoy into classroom activities to increase motivation. Generate ideas for individual students, such as favorite characters, colors, games, and food preferences. Oscar's list might include Elmo (especially stickers and getting to hold an Elmo figu-

rine), green crayons for coloring, the purple carpet square during circle time, sitting next to Miss Linda during lunch, turning the light switch on or off when entering or leaving the classroom, stamps on his hand, M&Ms, red and pink jelly beans, graham crackers, and orange juice.

 Check out *Chapter 6* to learn more about using preference assessments to find out what motivates your students.

Throughout the manual, you will see examples of incorporating motivating items and activities into the classroom to increase student responding. For example, Oscar may be more motivated to read if a story relates to Elmo. Also observe which activities the class as a whole enjoys. When are your students the most engaged and attentive? What activities do they like? How might your behavior affect their engagement? You might discover that you can keep the attention of the majority of your students at a certain time of day (e.g., after morning recess), with a specific activity (e.g., arts and crafts or cooking), or when you are behaving in a novel manner (e.g., singing, being silly, or talking in a whisper).

Consider factors that help you maximize your students' attention during group instruction, to make the most of every opportunity.

In general, CPRT can be creatively used in almost any setting with a variety of activities to meet many types of student goals. As you become more comfortable with the components of CPRT and ways to apply them, you will be able to use CPRT strategically to help your students meet their goals.

Take a few minutes to make some notes about what activities and materials you think motivate the students in your classroom.

When Should I Use CPRT?

CPRT can be integrated throughout the day. CPRT can be used during small-group activities such as art and snack time, during larger-group activities such as circle time, during play outside on the playground, and during academic tasks. For example, if you are on the playground with your students, you can use CPRT to work on communication skills, counting, or taking turns with a small group while playing basketball.

To be most effective, you must maintain your students' attention through active engagement. You also need to minimize your own possible distractions, to ensure that you are able to follow through after presenting cues to your students. For these reasons, it is important that you recognize and take advantage of moments when you and your students will be able to focus on each other and the learning activity. Avoid using CPRT at times when you anticipate that there will be too much distraction.

When CPRT Isn't the Best Choice

Sometimes CPRT may not be the best intervention for a specific instructional goal, activity, setting, or student. Although CPRT is adaptable to many circumstances, some factors may make the intervention less successful. Each of these factors is described in more detail below.

- *There is no natural or direct reward associated with the goal or activity.* Some lessons will not easily lend themselves to CPRT strategies because they contain no natural or direct reward. For example, some teachers and parents report that CPRT may not work well for teaching self-help skills such as toilet training, hand washing, or toothbrushing because there is nothing about these activities a student enjoys. Others find that one aspect of a self-help routine, such as flushing the toilet, can motivate the student to complete the other steps of the routine (pulling down pants, sitting on toilet, etc.). Similarly, a student may dislike some routines or activities so much that materials she typically likes do not serve a reinforcing function in this particular situation. For example, a child may dislike brushing his teeth enough that even a favorite Elmo toothbrush does not make the activity more fun. In these situations, you may need to rely on other unrelated ways to motivate the child, such as giving the child a sticker after he successfully brushes his teeth. Before eliminating CPRT as a teaching tool for an activity or lesson, discuss possible rewarding items or activities related to the task with other staff and the student's parents. You may find that a student enjoys turning off the bathroom light (a naturally occurring reward) enough to encourage hand-washing behavior!

- *The motivating activity is not under your control.* Just as identifying rewards for your students is important, having control over these rewards allows you to effectively increase desirable student behavior. Sometimes the most interesting part of an activity happens to be something outside of your control. For example, you may want to teach your students to sit with peers at lunch, eat appropriately, and engage in basic conversation. One student may happily eat her tacos and fruit salad because you provide the reinforcement of a cookie at the end of the meal.

Another student may practice asking his peers questions and listening while they answer because you allow him to invite a friend back to the room to play computer games during recess. However, if a student is more interested in looking at the fluorescent lights in the cafeteria than in getting a cookie or playing computer games with a friend, you may have very little control over this student's lunchtime behavior because you cannot control access to the lights.

It is important that you identify what is likely to reinforce a student's behavior, and determine whether you have control over potential motivating items in the environment.

- *The student is making no progress after intensive use of CPRT strategies.* As with any teaching strategy, sometimes a student may not make progress with CPRT. If CPRT is being implemented correctly and consistently throughout the school day, and the student is not making measurable progress, you should consider other strategies.

 Take a look at *Chapter 6* to learn more about integrating CPRT with other strategies and ways to measure student progress.

Chapter Summary

CPRT is a naturalistic behavioral intervention that has clear research support for use with children with autism. Autism, a pervasive developmental disorder, requires teaching strategies that increase motivation and can be used across curriculum areas. CPRT capitalizes on students' motivation and teaches skills throughout the school day to encourage learning in many environments. It is fun, versatile, adaptable, and effective. CPRT can be used to teach communication, social, play, and academic skills, and can be integrated with other classroom strategies.

CPRT has been developed with teachers to include methods for meeting specific student goals, collecting data on student progress, and integrating CPRT with other interventions in the classroom. The current manual has been developed by a group of psychologists, researchers, teachers, and school administrators to address these issues because we believe that children with autism are best served by a collaborative community approach. We call this new method Classroom Pivotal Response Teaching, or CPRT, to highlight changes that make the program more suited to classroom environments. The procedures described in this manual have been tested in real classrooms. We hope that this manual will help you use CPRT effectively in your unique classroom environment.

CHAPTER 2

Laying the Foundation
for CPRT

CHAPTER OVERVIEW

Applied Behavior Analysis (ABA) is the scientific study of the links between human behavior and the environment. Each behavior is preceded by an antecedent and followed by a consequence, which affects the likelihood that a specific behavior will occur again in the future. Understanding behavioral principles will help you learn CPRT because the foundations of CPRT are in ABA. The aim of ABA is to systematically evaluate and change human behavior in a positive way.

The following sections are included:

Learning Your ABCs: The Pattern of Behavior

Antecedents
    Using Verbal Cues
    Using Nonverbal Cues
    Hierarchy of Opportunities to Respond

Behavior
    Appropriate Response
    Reasonable Attempts at Appropriate Responding
    Inappropriate Response
    Incorrect Response

Consequences
    Consequences That Increase Behavior
    Consequences That Decrease Behavior
    Important Points to Remember about Consequences

What ABA Is *Not*

How ABA Relates to CPRT

Preparing to Use CPRT

This chapter has a corresponding training lecture on the DVD accompanying this manual (*CPRT Session 1: Learning Your ABCs*).

CPRT is based on the principles of **Applied Behavior Analysis (ABA)**. If you are not already familiar with ABA, this chapter provides a basic understanding of the principles used to develop CPRT. It is important to understand the applicability of ABA principles in the classroom before learning the specific steps of CPRT.

Learning the foundations will improve your use of CPRT and enhance your problem solving skills when using this approach.

Although parts of this chapter are somewhat technical and detailed, gaining a clear understanding of these principles will help you implement CPRT. The principles of ABA are the starting point for all behavioral interventions for children with autism. This chapter will also give you a head start in becoming familiar with the wide array of other behavioral interventions designed for children with autism.

 For more information about ABA, see *www.abainternational.org*; *Applied Behavior Analysis for Teachers* by Paul Alberto and Anne Troutman (2009); and *Understanding Applied Behavior Analysis* by Albert Kearney (2008).

Learning Your ABCs: The Pattern of Behavior

The term **behavioral interventions** refers to techniques developed by the science of ABA (see Table 2.5 for a detailed description). Although there are some differences in the exact teaching techniques of specific behavioral interventions, all such interventions adhere to an **operant model**. The word **operant** refers to the idea that learning is

the result of the consequences that follow a behavior, and these consequences determine how and how often a behavior is likely to occur in the future. In this chapter, you will learn how the operant model is related to the behavior of students with autism, though the same model can be applied equally well to any type of behavior.

An operant model consists of three main components: (1) an **antecedent** event, or an experience that happens before a behavior; (2) a **behavior**, or a response by a student (or lack of response, in some cases); and (3) a **consequence**, which serves to increase, decrease, or maintain the occurrence, duration, or intensity of the behavior in the future. This is called a **three-part contingency**, and it is illustrated in *Figure 2.1*. The three-part contingency is often referred to as the **ABC pattern of behavior**, in which A stands for antecedent, B for behavior, and C for consequence. The following is an introduction to the three parts of the contingency.

1. *Antecedent.* The antecedent is the event or experience that happens before the behavior. An opportunity to respond begins with a signal to the student, and can take many forms. The antecedent can be a verbal opportunity, such as a question or instruction, or a nonverbal opportunity, such as the presence of an object in the environment (e.g., a toy, a fire engine, a peer, a time of day). (See *Antecedents*, below, for more information on types of antecedents.) As adults, we behave under the control of antecedent signals all the time. Our behavior is controlled by such antecedents as the color of a traffic signal, a question from a child, the time on a clock, or the feeling of hunger. A signal in the environment controls behavior because it promises certain consequences for responding (or not responding).

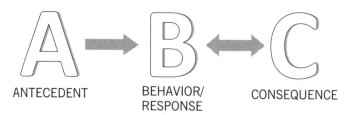

FIGURE 2.1. **Three-Part Contingency.** These are the three components of the operant model.

2. *Behavior.* The behavior is the response from your student that you want to increase, decrease, or maintain. The behavior follows the antecedent. Our behavior in response to the presence of a red traffic signal (antecedent), for example, is to hit the brakes (behavior). In the classroom, your student performs some sort of response to an opportunity (antecedent) that is either going to be appropriate, inappropriate, incorrect, or an approximation of a correct response. Also, your student might make no response. (See *Behavior*, below, for more information on types of responses.)

3. *Consequence.* The consequence is your response to your student's behavior. This is an extremely important part of the pattern. There are consequences that will increase the strength of the behavior, those that will maintain the behavior, and still other consequences that will decrease the strength of the behavior. These types of consequences are discussed in detail in this chapter. The consequence of successfully passing a spelling test, for example, maintains the behavior of studying (see *Table 2.1*). Consequences are most effective when they are delivered immediately after the behavior and are contingent (i.e., dependent) on the behavior.

Now let's look at each of these parts in more detail.

TABLE 2.1. ABC Example

This table illustrates how the same antecedent (a spelling test) can lead to different behaviors, consequences, and results.

Antecedent	Behavior	Consequence	Result
Your student has a spelling test on Tuesday.	Your student studies for the spelling test.	Your student gets a good grade on the test.	Your student is likely to study next time she has a test. (Increase in positive behavior)
	Your student plays computer games instead of studying for the spelling test.	Your student fails the spelling test.	Your student is more likely to study for the next test. (Increase in positive behavior)
		Your student gets a good grade on the test.	Your student is more likely to play computer games instead of studying next time she has a test. (Increase in negative behavior)

Antecedents

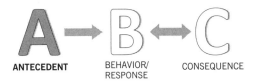

There are many ways to create opportunities for your student to use her communication, play, social, and academic skills. These **opportunities to respond** (also called **cues**) will act as antecedents for behavior. The type of opportunities you use should be based on your student's skill level and should be varied throughout an extended interaction with your student. Using a variety of clear opportunities to respond will help your student generalize what she has learned to new environments and people. If the opportunity you present is too difficult for the student to understand or if she is unable to respond, you can provide a more concrete opportunity to help her remain successful.

Opportunities to respond are often confused with **prompts**. An opportunity to respond, or cue, is the first presentation of a signal for a student to engage in a behavior, action, or reply. A prompt is the subsequent support you provide a student to ensure a successful response to the opportunity presented if he is having trouble. This relationship is highlighted in *Figure 2.2.* For example, by holding up a pencil and looking expectantly at your student, you present an opportunity to respond. If your student does not communicate with you to ask for the pencil, you can provide a prompt by saying, "Pencil." We next describe specific ways to present opportunities for responding.

Opportunity to Respond
• The first presentation of a signal for a student to engage in a behavior, action, or reply, or an environmental arrangement that encourages spontaneous responding.
Prompt
• The subsequent support you provide to a student to ensure a successful response to the opportunity presented if she is having trouble.

FIGURE 2.2. Opportunity to Respond versus Prompt. This figure highlights the difference between the first opportunity to respond you provide your student and the prompts you may give to help support that response.

Using Verbal Cues

There are several ways of presenting an opportunity to respond by using language or verbal communication. Students who are just learning to communicate are likely to respond to more simple cues, such as providing a verbal model or instruction, while students with more advanced communication skills should respond to questions or comments.

Verbal Model (Exact or Open-Ended)

Providing a sound, word, or phrase as a verbal model is a simple way to encourage a student response. You can encourage your student to give a verbal response by clearly labeling the object or activity that interests the student. A verbal model can be *exactly* what you want the student to say, such as "Push car," or a cue to elicit a response, such as "Push … [expecting *car*]."

Instruction

Sometimes you want to encourage a nonverbal behavior from the student that is best communicated directly. You can provide a direct instruction, such as "Feed the doll," "Throw away the trash," or "Sit down, please."

Question

Presenting a question is another good way to encourage a student response. Responding to the question requires that the student understands your question and that she possesses the skills to respond verbally or nonverbally without a model. You can ask your student a direct question, such as "Do you want to do math or reading?", "What do you want?", or "How many balls do you want?" Avoid overly complex or indirect questions, such as "Should we put two balls or three balls down the ramp really fast?" (see *Component 2: Clear and Appropriate Instruction* in *Chapter 3*). It is easy to get in the habit of asking questions. However, it is important to use other methods of presenting opportunities as well, so that your student can begin to verbalize without being asked a direct question. Too many questions in a row can also be stressful for some students and thus may make them likely to disengage from the interaction.

Comment

As your student's skills develop, you might comment on a situation to encourage a response. This is more difficult than the verbal cues described above, so you should be sure to simplify language if needed, and to confirm that your student is attending to you when you use this method. For example, you might make a comment that extends an activity. Saying, "I see that you finished your worksheet; the reading corner is open," may encourage your student to initiate a request to read independently.

> *Use comments instead of questions whenever possible to encourage spontaneous responding.*

Using Nonverbal Cues

Providing a nonverbal behavior such as pointing, signing, modeling, or gesturing is a simple way to encourage a response. Nonverbal behaviors can allow a student an opportunity to spontaneously produce a specific behavior, or can provide a very directive opportunity to respond. A nonverbal model may accompany a verbal model as well.

Gesture or Play Action

Your student can learn more complex communication or play skills by watching you use a specific gesture or play in a new way with a toy. You can model pointing to an item your student would like, and then help your student imitate the point to obtain the item. If your student wants to play with alphabet blocks by putting them in a cup, you can model a new functional play skill. You might take a block and stack it on another block, then have your student do the same, followed by free access to the blocks. This is also a wonderful way to expand imaginative play. For example, if your student likes to roll cars back and forth, you (or a peer) can model putting a car down a ramp, putting gas in a car, or parking the car in a garage. Requiring your student to imitate one of the novel actions with the car, before allowing the student to roll the car back and forth, can encourage new play behaviors. Similarly, modeling activities such as drawing, cutting, completing worksheets, and the like can help students who respond well to visual cues.

Facial Expression (Expectant Waiting)

To encourage spontaneous communication, it is important that you do not speak every time you want a student to say something. Constantly providing verbal cues to your student may teach her to rely on a cue from you instead of generating her own sounds and words spontaneously. Using an expectant facial expression (eyes wide and eyebrows lifted) will also help your student understand social cues. This is called **expectant waiting**. For example, while singing a song your student enjoys, you can stop in mid-song and wait for him to indicate that you should keep going. If your student comes to a cabinet in search of markers, you can block the door and look expectantly toward your student for the word "help" or "markers." After several seconds, add a gestural prompt, comment, question, or instruction to assist the student if necessary. Expectant waiting is a technique that is appropriate whenever the student understands what is expected.

Situational

Sometimes naturally occurring situations arise that may promote communication or other behavior. For example, your student may need to ask for your help to open the door to go outside, or for a friend's help to get a bike out of a shed. You can also set up activities or situations that are incomplete, in order to elicit communication or social initiations from your student. These are sometimes called **communicative tempta-** **tions**. Place toys or snacks out of reach so that your student needs to ask for your assistance, or give a small amount of a snack to encourage her to ask for more. You may put out a worksheet, but leave the pencil out of reach so that the student needs to ask for it to begin. Blocking access to natural reinforcers is a useful way to provide incentives for your student to initiate.

Hierarchy of Opportunities to Respond

When using CPRT, you will vary the types of opportunities you present. For example, you may begin with a situational opportunity by just making a toy available (e.g., leaving a toy garage near the cars your student often lines up). Your student may respond by putting a car in the garage. If your student does not respond to the situation you have presented (and he is not likely to in the beginning), you may structure the interaction more by commenting, "The garage is empty. It needs a car." Alternatively, you may know that a specific student is not yet able to respond to this type of opportunity. Instead, you could provide a model (saying, "Car in," and driving a car into the garage), followed by an instruction to the student ("Car in"). The particular opportunity you provide will depend on your student and the situation.

Table 2.2 presents a hierarchy of opportunities to respond—that is, types of cues ranked from least to most difficult. If a student consistently needs a high level of prompting to respond to your cues, it may be helpful to move back a level in the type of opportunity you present. Alternatively, if a student is consistently responding independently and spontaneously, you should consider moving up a level to increase the difficulty of your cues.

TABLE 2.2. Hierarchy of Opportunities to Respond

A teacher is working with a student to teach the play skill of feeding a doll. Depending on the student's current level of play ability, the teacher will choose different opportunities to encourage the student to respond.

	Type of opportunity	Definition	Example
Decreasing levels of support	Gesture/play model	Model the action expected from the student.	Hold up a toy and model a point. Feed a doll with a spoon.
	Verbal model (exact or open-ended)	Model a sound or word for the student to imitate, or provide the first part of a familiar phrase for the student to complete.	Say, "Spoon," when the student is reaching for the spoon.
	Instruction	Give a direct instruction telling the student exactly what to do.	Say, "Feed the boy."
	Question	Ask a direct question for your student to answer. The level of support varies with the type of question (e.g., requiring a choice among options vs. open-ended).	Say, "Should the boy eat peas or yogurt?"
	Facial expression	Wait expectantly while attending to the student. Lift your eyebrows and open your eyes wide while controlling access to desired materials or activities.	Hold up the doll and give your student an expectant look.
	Comment	Make a leading comment when your student is attending to you.	Gain the student's attention and say, "The boy is hungry."
	Situational	Set up activities or situations that are incomplete or broken to elicit communication.	Put a doll, spoon, and bowl on the table near the student.

Behavior

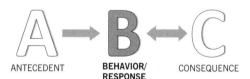

Once you have presented an opportunity to respond, the next step is to observe your student's behavior in response to that opportunity. How your student responds will determine what you do next, so it is important to watch closely. Observing your student will help you react to her behavior quickly and accurately.

Because CPRT is a naturalistic intervention, you will often present opportunities to respond that do not require one specific response. Consider how you would naturally greet a friend or coworker. You could say,

"Hello!"; ask, "How are you?"; wave enthusiastically; give a hug; or nod toward the person. In the same way, there are multiple ways for your student to respond appropriately. Expecting, prompting, or rewarding the same response from your student over many opportunities may promote rote communication, play, and social skills. Instead, reward a variety of responses to promote generalization, and encourage your student to learn a broader range of appropriate behavior. It may be helpful to think of responses in terms of appropriate or inappropriate rather than correct or incorrect, to keep in mind that you are expecting a general type of response rather than an exact action, expression, or behavior.

After observing your student's response, you must decide whether it is an appropriate or inappropriate reply to the opportunity you have presented. Several factors, including environment, activity, student ability, and target skill, determine the appropriateness of your student's response. The different types of responses your student may give are discussed in more detail in this section.

Appropriate Response

Any student response that you wish to occur more frequently in the future should be considered appropriate. When a student responds with a positive communicative, play, social, or academic answer, you will reward the behavior (see *Consequences That Increase Behavior*).

An appropriate response is any behavior from the student that falls within the range of skills you are targeting in an interaction.

The type of opportunity you present determines the appropriateness of a response. If you present a cue in a question form that calls for a yes–no answer (e.g., "Can I have a turn?"), your student may respond by saying, "No." Although this is certainly not the response you had in mind, it is an appropriate response, given the cue presented. Similarly, if you ask your student, "What do you want?" and he responds, "All done," this is a logical answer to your question. It may be necessary to present more targeted cues (e.g., "It's my turn now!" or "What worksheet do you want?" in the examples just given), in order to ensure that you get the type of response you want from your student.

An appropriate response for one student may not be appropriate for another student. For example, it may be appropriate for a pre-verbal student to place an adult's hand on a closed container as a way to ask to have the container opened, but this same action may not be appropriate from a student who is working on verbalizations. Since it is likely that the students in your classroom are at various skill levels, it is important to consider the behavior you observe in the context of each student's current abilities.

If a student is responding appropriately and independently to nearly all of the cues presented, it may be an indication that you can increase the difficulty of your cue or target a more complex response. Such adjustments should be made slowly with close monitoring of student motivation, to ensure continued student involvement in the activity.

Reasonable Attempts at Appropriate Responding

In CPRT, it is important to identify reasonable **attempts** at appropriate behavior, even if a response does not reflect a student's full ability. For example, if a student who has clearly articulated "ball" in the past instead uses the sound "buh" to request a ball, this would be considered an attempt. If a student who is learning to play functionally with a puzzle puts a piece on the puzzle board but cannot rotate it correctly to fit into its place, this would also be considered an attempt. It is important to be aware of the student's current skill level in order to determine what constitutes an attempt. You should require the attempt to be goal-directed, meaning (1) that it serves the same function as the skill you are targeting and is only slightly less accurate or complex, and (2) that it is within the student's ability (i.e., the student is clearly trying). It is important to balance an acceptance of reasonable attempts with high expectations for new skill acquisition. This balance is discussed further, and more examples of appropriate attempts are provided, in *Component 8: Reinforcement of Attempts* in *Chapter 3.*

An attempt is a behavior that serves the same function as the target skill, without the accuracy or complexity of a "correct" response.

Inappropriate Response

It is likely that students will fail to respond appropriately some of the time. Inappropriate behaviors are unrelated to the interaction (e.g., self-stimulatory behaviors, talking about an item/topic not related to the teaching activity) or disruptive to the teaching environment (e.g., crying, yelling, running away). The absence of a response is also part of this category. When your student responds inappropriately, deliver a consequence that is designed to decrease the future occurrence of that response (see *Consequences That Decrease Behavior*).

A seemingly appropriate response may in fact be inappropriate if it is coupled with extraneous or negative behaviors. A student who is answering a question and engaging in the self-stimulatory behavior of waving her hands in front of her face at the same time is not responding appropriately. If this combination of behaviors is reinforced, it may be difficult for her to determine which of her behaviors is being rewarded. Similarly, a nonverbal student who is rewarded with going outside after gesturing toward the door through tears may learn that crying gets the door open. Watch for superfluous behaviors accompanying the desired response, to make sure you are rewarding only the responses you wish to increase.

Incorrect Response

Finally, a student may simply respond incorrectly. For example, if you ask, "What color is this crayon?" and hold up a red crayon, but the student responds, "Blue," this is not correct. Even if the student is trying and attending, you should not reward incorrect responses. For quick reference, *Table 2.3* summarizes the various ways your student may react to the opportunity you present.

Incorrect responses may indicate a lack of attention or motivation, or the need to provide additional prompts to teach the student the correct response.

TABLE 2.3. Types of Behavioral Responses

Students may exhibit a variety of responses to your cues. Here are some examples.

Response	Description	Example
Appropriate response	Falls within the range of skills you are targeting.	Follows instruction to pick up pieces; says, "One more time, please!"
Reasonable attempt	Serves the same function as the target skill, without the same accuracy or complexity.	Says, "Please!" to indicate he wants to keep playing.
Inappropriate response	Unrelated to the interaction or disruptive; failure to respond.	Yells, "No!" and grabs the shapes.
Incorrect response	Incorrect.	Picks up red pieces after you tell him to pick up blue pieces.

Consequences

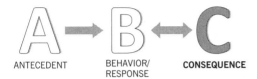

ANTECEDENT   BEHAVIOR/   CONSEQUENCE
              RESPONSE

A consequence follows a student's behavior and either increases or decreases the likelihood that the student will behave that way in the future.

Consequences That Increase Behavior

Positive reinforcement refers to presenting an event or item that increases the likelihood that the behavior it follows will happen again. Typically this means presenting something your student likes only when the desired behavior occurs. This will increase the strength of the behavior that the reinforcer follows. For example, following an appropriate behavior with giving your student a favored toy, providing praise, or offering a desired food item is likely to serve as positive reinforcement, and therefore that behavior is more likely to occur again in the future.

Negative reinforcement refers to the removal after a behavior of a situation or object your student does not like, which increases the likelihood of the behavior's occurring in the future. Behaviors maintained by negative reinforcement are often called **escape behaviors** or **avoidance behaviors**, because the motive to continue the behavior is the likelihood of escaping or avoiding a nonpreferred experience. For example, a child throws a tantrum when she is required to eat dinner at the table rather than in front of the television. Her parents can respond to the behavior by requiring her to stay at the table or by allowing her to avoid the table. If her parents decide to let her eat dinner in front of the television after

she throws a tantrum at the table, the child's tantrums are likely to increase in the future because she can escape the undesired activity of sitting at the table by having a tantrum.

However, negative reinforcement is not always negative! In fact, you can use this strategy to increase your students' appropriate behavior. For example, you may allow a student who dislikes sitting at his desk to leave his chair once he finishes a writing assignment. He is reinforced for finishing his work by being allowed to escape the nonpreferred situation of sitting at his desk, and therefore he is more likely to finish his work in the future.

Consequences That Decrease Behavior

Punishment occurs when a behavior is followed by an event or experience that your student dislikes, thus decreasing the likelihood of the behavior's occurring in the future. For instance, during art, your student throws crayons on the floor, and you require her to pick them up. If picking the crayons up is something your student does not like to do, then the throwing behavior will decrease. Similarly, if your student does not like to hear the word "no," then saying "no" when she does something inappropriate should reduce that behavior. (It is important to point out that "no" is also often used as an informational word, and may not be a punisher in many situations.) Punishers are everywhere in our environment and serve to discourage dangerous or inappropriate behaviors. A child who touches a hot stove and gets burned is certainly less likely to touch a hot stove in the future, because the behavior of touching the stove has been followed by punishment.

There is another form of punishment used to decrease a behavior. This second type of punishment occurs when your student's behavior results in the loss of positive reinforcement. This is referred to as **response cost**, or, more commonly, **time away**. If your student is disruptive in the classroom, you may place him in another location where he cannot have access to the fun and interesting things in the classroom. (Of course, remember that time away is only effective if the time in environment is rewarding and preferable to the student.) Another good example of the response cost form of punishment is the loss of privileges, such as access to a computer or TV.

Extinction is a third way to decrease behavior. Extinction occurs when a behavior is no longer followed by a consequence that maintained it previously. Consider a case where a bully likes to tease another student. The bully enjoys the student's reaction to the teasing and so constantly seeks out the student to tease her again. If the student ignores the bully and no longer reacts to the bully's comments, then the positive consequence (the student's reaction to teasing) is no longer reinforcing the teasing behavior, and the bully will stop. In another example, if your student has learned to get your attention by making inappropriate noises, you are likely to reduce this behavior by no longer attending to it. You are extinguishing the inappropriate noise behavior by no longer following it with a positive consequence (your attention). It is important to know that when you are using extinction, it is likely that the student's disruptive behavior will increase before it gets better. This is called an **extinction burst** and can actually mean that what you are doing is working. Take the example of a student making inappropriate noises. Making those noises successfully got your attention quickly for a long time. When the noises suddenly don't work any more, the student is likely to try harder to get your attention by making louder noises or different noises. It is important to continue to put the behavior on extinction as it

increases, in order to be sure it will go away completely. Teaching another, more appropriate behavior (e.g., raising a hand) is also helpful, so that your student can replace the inappropriate behavior with an appropriate one that has the same function (getting your attention).

Important Points to Remember about Consequences

When we talk about punishment, we are talking about an event or experience that is undesirable or nonpreferred to the student. Nothing about the types of punishment discussed here denotes pain or harm. A punisher is any event or experience that the student does not like and that serves to decrease the behavior it follows. Punishment can be a frown, looking away, a nonpreferred task, or a statement of disappointment. Corporal punishment that involves touching or harming a student in any way should not be used in the classroom.

The type of consequence is defined solely by the effect the event has on student behavior.

Events or experiences that seem positive (e.g., a toy, playing outside, a piece of candy) may in fact be punishers and decrease the behavior they follow, depending on the student. For example, if you hold up a noisemaker toy in front of your student during free play and give an expectant look (antecedent), the student may point to the toy (behavior) and receive the item in response to this request (consequence). It may be tempting to assume that because toys are generally a preferred item, receiving a toy in response to the pointing behavior will increase the occurrence of this behavior in the future. However, if the student activates the toy and finds the noises or music it makes unpleasant (e.g., too loud, too fast), then that toy may actually be a punisher, because the student may be less likely to point to toys in the future in order to avoid a similar unpleasant experience. Alternatively, experiences that seem negative (e.g., receiving a verbal reprimand, being required to pick up thrown crayons) may in fact be reinforcers and therefore increase the behavior they follow. Time away is the most common example of this. If your student is disruptive during math because she doesn't like to do math, then receiving time away during math will actually increase the disruptive behavior, because time away allows the student to escape from the demand of doing the assignment. In other words, the time away is actually a reinforcer in this case, because the student is more likely to be disruptive during math in the future to avoid the task again. It is important to define consequences by their effect on behavior, and not use general conceptions of experiences or events (e.g., candy = good, time away = bad) to determine whether something is a

reinforcer or a punisher. See *Table 2.4* for examples of each of the different ways to respond to student behavior.

What ABA Is *Not*

Although popular vernacular often uses "applied behavior analysis" or "ABA" to describe a specific type of behavioral intervention, this is inaccurate. When people refer to the intervention received by a child with autism as ABA, they are typically thinking of a specific, highly structured form of behavioral teaching more properly referred to as Discrete Trial Teaching (DTT; see *Chapters 1 and 6*). This misunderstanding and misuse of the term ABA hinders the ability of service providers and parents to fully appreciate the magnitude of ABA and utilize its enduring principles. ABA is a type of scientific inquiry characterized by certain research designs and principles (see *Table 2.5*); it is not a specific treatment for children with autism. In fact, ABA is the foundation for interventions for a wide variety of indi-

---

TABLE 2.4. Types of Consequences

A teacher is working with two students to complete a puzzle. They have to share the puzzle pieces and board. One of the students is getting frustrated and says, "It's my turn," in a somewhat whiney voice. This table demonstrates how the teacher could respond in several different ways, depending on how she wants to affect the student's behavior in the future.

Type of consequence	Description	Example
Positive reinforcement	Presentation of a desired item after a behavior, which leads to an increase in the behavior.	Give student the puzzle for a turn.
Negative reinforcement	Removal of an undesirable situation or item after a behavior, which leads to an increase in the behavior.	Remove other student from activity so the student no longer has to share the puzzle.
Punishment	Presentation of an undesirable situation or item after a behavior, which leads to a decrease in the behavior.	Take puzzle away from student.
Extinction	Discontinuation of reinforcement, which leads to a decrease in the behavior.	Allow the other student to keep playing with the puzzle.

viduals to address an even wider variety of behaviors. For example, research involving ABA focuses on a range of topics, including (but by no means limited to) how to get teenagers to wear seatbelts, college students to study effectively, and elderly nursing home residents to use leisure time well.

ABA is not a specific type of teaching for children with autism or any other individuals.

TABLE 2.5. What Is ABA?

ABA is the study of the relationship between human behavior and the environment, or linking how events and experiences in our environment shape patterns of future behavior. The task of ABA is to understand the laws governing how the environment affects behavior, and to use these laws to change behavior in a positive manner. This table provides a technical overview of the entirety of ABA, as well as the criteria a scientific inquiry must fulfill in order to fall in this category.

Criteria	Explanation	Example
Applied	Address problems of social significance and provide direct benefit to people's lives.	Studying how to structure the environment to help a child with autism eat a more varied diet.
Behavioral	Examine how to get an individual to do something (or stop doing something). Scientific study of these matters requires precise, objective measurement.	Investigating how to get a child to expand her play skills (do something) and specifying a measurable, objective goal, such as "Engages with 4 toys in 20 minutes."
Analytic	Use a specific set of research designs that clearly identify when changes in behavior are caused by specific manipulations, not by chance.	Research designs are most commonly single-subject designs where individual participants are carefully studied.
Technological	Identify and describe the techniques making up a particular intervention with enough detail for others to implement the intervention and achieve the same results.	A technological description of CPRT specifies the required steps as defined in this manual.
Conceptually systematic	Describe teaching strategies in terms of general principles, and interpret results in terms of the concepts from which they were derived.	Labeling the statement, "Nice sitting quietly, Denise!" as "social reinforcement" identifies the phrase as part of a conceptual system.
Effective	Evaluate effectiveness on the basis of practical value and social significance.	An intervention that can reduce the self-injurious behavior of head hitting from 100 times a day to 15 times is useful, but not practically valuable. The intervention must eliminate the self-injurious behavior in order to meet this criterion.
Generality	Demonstrate that a change in behavior affected by an intervention is durable over time (maintenance), appears in a wide variety of environments (stimulus generalization), and/or spreads to a wide variety of related behaviors (response generalization).	A student is said to have learned to read sight words if he can do so a week after the lesson, at home and/ or in a book. Also, you would expect similar, untaught words to emerge in the student's reading vocabulary.

Note. See Baer, Wolf, and Risley (1968) for further details.

How ABA Relates to CPRT

Because CPRT is based on the principles of ABA, a basic understanding of these concepts is important for successful CPRT implementation. The specific components of CPRT are based on the ABC pattern described in this chapter and are discussed in *Chapter 3*. You will first learn about presenting an opportunity to respond, which corresponds to the antecedent. You will learn strategies for providing different types of opportunities to your student and for setting up the environmental context for a successful interaction. Next you will learn how to observe your student's responses, as well as the various types of behaviors your student might use. Finally, you will learn about responding to the student, which corresponds to the consequence. You will learn important strategies for using specific types of consequences that will assist your student in better understanding the relationships between her actions and the environment.

Preparing to Use CPRT

As you continue to learn about CPRT, you can prepare to use the intervention with your students. Maximizing your students' motivation is an essential part of using CPRT. For this reason, it is important to have a good understanding of what motivates your specific students. You may know of some items or activities that all students enjoy, but typically students will have individual preferences and interests. We recommend that you use two primary techniques to identify what motivates your students. First, gather information from other people who know your students well. Parents, former teachers, and other service providers will have valuable information on what techniques and tools they have used to motivate your students.

We have included a *Gathering Information* worksheet in this manual to be distributed for this purpose. You can see a completed example of the *Gathering Information* worksheet in *Chapter 6* (see *Figure 6.3*), and a blank copy of this form is provided as *Handout 3* in *Part IV* of the manual. Next, conduct your own assessment of your students' preferred materials and activities. A **preference assessment** is a formal and systematic way of gathering information on what a student enjoys. We have described two methods of conducting a preference assessment later in this manual. Please refer to *Chapter 6* to see a full description of how to conduct each type of preference assessment; *Figures 6.4 and 6.5* are completed examples of the two accompanying forms. Blank copies of both forms are provided as *Handouts 4 and 5* in *Part IV*.

Keep your students' motivation in mind as you continue to read. Think about your students, their interests, and how you currently run your classroom as you read through the CPRT components in *Chapter 3*. This will help prepare you to integrate CPRT into your daily work.

Chapter Summary

CPRT is based on the principles of ABA, and it is important to understand these principles in order to utilize CPRT accurately and flexibly. ABA is not a specific treatment for children with autism; instead, it is the study of the relationship between human behavior and the environment. Like other behavioral interventions, CPRT is based on an operant model, also called the ABC pattern of behavior. In CPRT, an antecedent is the opportunity to respond that you present your student. There are several verbal and nonverbal ways to present a cue to respond to your student, with varying degrees of difficulty. The behavior is how your student responds to the opportunity you present. In CPRT, a student's behavior may be considered an appropriate and correct response, a good attempt, an inappropriate response, or an incorrect response. A consequence is the response you provide to your student's behavior. The type of consequence that follows a behavior determines how likely that behavior is to occur again in the future. Once you understand the ABC pattern of behavior, it is important to identify motivating materials for your student, so that you can effectively reinforce desired skills.

CHAPTER 3

Components of CPRT
Using CPRT with Individual Students

CHAPTER OVERVIEW

CPRT involves presenting an opportunity to the student (antecedent), observing the student's response (behavior), and responding to the student's behavior (consequence). Each of these behavioral elements can be broken down into specific components, which are the strategies you can use when interacting with your students. This chapter describes each of the eight components in detail and provides the foundational information you will need to implement CPRT.

The following sections are included:

Set the Stage: Antecedent Strategies
    Component 1: Student Attention
    Component 2: Clear and Appropriate Instruction
    Component 3: Easy and Difficult Tasks (Maintenance/Acquisition)
    Component 4: Shared Control (Student Choice/Turn Taking)
    Component 5: Multiple Cues (Broadening Attention)

Watch What Happens: Student Behavior

React: Consequence Strategies
    Component 6: Direct Reinforcement
    Component 7: Contingent Consequence (Immediate and Appropriate)
    Component 8: Reinforcement of Attempts

This chapter has a corresponding training lecture on the DVD accompanying this manual (*CPRT Session 2: The Components of CPRT*).

Now that you have an understanding of the behavioral foundations of CPRT, it's time to learn about the specific components of the intervention. There are eight components of CPRT, and they can be thought of in terms of antecedent strategies and consequence strategies.

Set the Stage: Antecedent Strategies

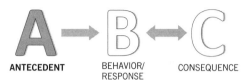

ANTECEDENT   BEHAVIOR/ RESPONSE   CONSEQUENCE

As described in *Chapter 2*, antecedent strategies (the ways you set up the environment for a student to respond) help you teach new skills, motivate students, and encourage generalization and initiation. Antecedent strategies are also known as cues or opportunities to respond. The type of opportunity or cue you present to your student will depend on the student's skill level and the learning activity. Keep in mind that cues can be presented verbally or nonverbally, and look back at the *Antecedents* section of *Chapter 2* for a full review of the types of cues. A brief summary of antecedent types is provided in *Table 3.1*. CPRT Components 1, 2, 3, 4, and 5 involve the effective presentation of these cues or opportunities to respond.

COMPONENT 1: STUDENT ATTENTION

Be sure your student is paying attention before you ask him to do or say something.

Attention refers to where a student is directing his focus. Students with autism seem to pay too little attention to important stimuli (e.g., a teacher's instruction) and too much attention to the "wrong" stimuli in their environment (e.g., a spinning fan or the wheels of a car). Therefore, Component 1 of CPRT states that you should be sure your student is attending to what you are doing or saying before providing an opportunity to respond. You may need to actively gain your student's attention; otherwise, it will be impossible for your student to respond correctly. If your student is paying attention, he is more likely to understand instructions and become engaged in the activity. Over time, increasing attention to toys, activity, and people will lead to increased and extended engagement through play and conversation. It will also improve all your students' ability to pay attention in a group.

TABLE 3.1. Types of Antecedents: Opportunities to Respond

This table lists antecedents in order from most to least support for the student.

	Type of opportunity	Definition
Decreasing levels of support ↓	Gesture/play model	Model the action expected from the student.
	Verbal model (exact or open-ended)	Model a sound or word for the student to imitate, or provide the first part of a familiar phrase for the student to complete.
	Instruction	Give a direct instruction telling the student exactly what to do.
	Question	Ask a direct question for your student to answer. The level of support varies with the type of question (e.g., requiring a choice among options vs. open-ended).
	Facial expression	Wait expectantly while attending to the student. Lift your eyebrows and open your eyes wide while controlling access to desired materials or activities.
	Comment	Make a leading comment when your student is attending to you.
	Situational cues	Set up activities or situations that are incomplete or broken to elicit communication.

If you are having difficulty engaging your student in an opportunity to respond, you may need to provide more structured opportunities (verbal model, instruction) before moving to more advanced types of opportunities (expectant waiting, situational cues, etc.).

A student with autism may struggle to maintain her attention to a teacher or activity, or may attend to you in a way that is unusual. For example, although eye contact is a primary way to communicate attention, a student with autism may find it difficult to make or maintain eye contact with you. While your student is learning to make eye contact, you should rely on other behaviors that indicate she is attending to you. These behaviors include body orientation (turning her body toward you), reaching, pointing, imitating your actions or sounds, attending to the desired object, or looking at you out of the corner of her eye. *Figure 3.1* highlights common indicators of attention. You should identify which behaviors indicate attention for individual students.

Possible Indicators of Attention

- Student is looking toward the teacher (maybe out of the corner of the eye).
- Student is looking toward the teaching materials.
- Student's body is oriented toward the teacher or materials.
- Student is not engaged in self-stimulatory behavior.
- Student is not actively engaged with another object.
- Student is reaching for teaching materials or toy.

FIGURE 3.1. **Possible Indicators of Attention.** There are many ways a student with autism may indicate attention.

It is also important to identify behaviors that indicate inattention for your students. Sometimes it is clear that a student is not attending. For example, behaviors such as crying, yelling, and engaging in verbal or nonverbal stereotypic or self-stimulatory behavior (e.g., hand flapping) all indicate that your student may not be attending. Other behaviors may be more difficult to interpret. A student who is facing you but holding a preferred toy, or one who is sitting next to you at a table but staring up toward the corner, may or may not be attending to you. In these situations, you should rely on your knowledge of the student and use a cue to assess or gain his attention.

There are several methods you can use to increase the likelihood that your student will pay attention to you.

Choose Motivating Activities

It is important to use toys and activities that your student enjoys. Language, play, social, and academic skills can be taught using almost anything! Your student may enjoy puzzles or race cars and can ask for those using sounds, words, or phrase speech. A block might be used initially to teach constructive play or word imitation, and later as a "cookie" for teaching symbolic play. Even activities that seem to elicit self-stimulatory or stereotyped behavior may be motivating. For example, if your student enjoys watching fans spin, he might ask to turn it on, spin it faster, or pretend it is an airplane engine.

 Providing manipulatives during circle time, such as figurines, squishy balls, or sock puppets, is great way to maintain student attention and interest in the activity.

If your student enjoys physical activity, he can ask to spin in a chair or bounce on a ball. These objects and activities can be used for teaching even if your student is not using them appropriately. If your student enjoys messy play, try sand, shaving cream, or finger paints. To help identify motivating activities, observe what the student chooses to do when left on her own and conduct a preference assessment. The idea is that your student will be motivated to engage with you and pay attention when she enjoys the objects and activities you are using.

 Check out the *Identifying Motivating Materials* section of *Chapter 6* for a description of how to conduct a preference assessment to identify motivating materials for your students.

Be Close

Proximity is an important part of gaining attention. When you are going to provide an opportunity to your student, be sure you are nearby. Your student will be more likely to attend to an opportunity you provide from nearby than one you provide from across the room. Get down to your student's level so that eye contact is possible. If your student is sitting, sit with him. If your student is standing, but is very young, you may need to squat down in order to gain his attention. If it is the first instruction in the interaction, you may need to touch your student on the arm to gain his attention. Providing an opportunity for close face-to-face contact will help ensure that your student is able to attend to your instructions and be successful in responding. It may be helpful to begin using CPRT in a smaller space if your student has great difficulty with attention and proximity. If you are in a group setting, try to have your students sit in a half-circle facing you. Some students may be able to sit

on the floor, while others may need the support of a chair or another adult in order to remain engaged.

 If your student is having difficulty paying attention during CPRT interactions, you may need to begin by expecting only brief periods of attention, and slowly increase your expectations as your student becomes successful.

Be Fun and Engaging

The more you enjoy yourself, the more your students will enjoy playing with you and listening to you. Although CPRT can be challenging in the beginning, once your students understand what you are expecting, you will all enjoy yourselves. Some students may respond better to a loud and silly teacher, while others may attend better to a calm, quiet voice and slow actions. As you get to know your students better, you will come to understand what level of animation and volume keeps them paying attention.

Be playful, silly, and animated, and watch your students' reaction to the things you do.

Keep It Natural

Gaining your student's attention in a natural way should eliminate the need to specifically teach attending skills. Try to avoid repeatedly calling the student's name or asking for attention (e.g., "Look at me"). These prompts will be difficult to eliminate if your student forms a habit of waiting for you to gain her attention. Instead, follow some of the suggestions listed above to encourage your student to attend naturally.

Build Tolerance for Attention
to the Teaching Activity

When you begin using CPRT, a student's attention span may be very short. To reduce frustration for both you and your student, begin by expecting only brief periods of attention. Short interactions can lead to longer interactions later. You may start with several brief exchanges throughout the school day. Then, increase your expectations as your student is able to attend for longer periods of time. This may lead to completing games, helping make a snack, singing complete songs, and telling stories together.

In *Table 3.2*, several scenarios are provided in which the teacher is providing a student with an opportunity to respond. Notice the likely difference in student response if the opportunity is provided when a student is paying attention versus when he is not.

TABLE 3.2. Attention: Examples			
This table provides examples of cue presentation with and without student attention across curriculum areas.			
Type	**Setting**	**Attention**	**Inattention**
Play	You are teaching Sam to follow one-step instructions during play. Sam is playing with cars in the play area.	You sit down in the play area facing Sam. You place your hand in front of Sam's car and wait until Sam looks at you. You then tell him, "Roll the car down." He follows the direction and gets to roll the wheels of the car.	You walk past the play area on your way to answer the phone and see Sam playing with cars. Since he is learning to follow one-step instructions, you say, "Sam, roll the car down." Sam does not acknowledge the instruction.
Language	Gabriella loves animals, and she is learning to use complete sentences to make requests. It is play time, and she is sitting in the reading area. You get several books about animals and walk over to the reading area.	You sit down so that you are on Gabriella's level and hold up the books. You wait until she has pointed to one of them, and you ask her, "What should we do?" She says, "Read the book," and you expand, "Let's read the penguin book," as you open the first page.	Standing in the reading area, you hold up the books and ask, "Which one should we read, Gabriella?" She does not respond, so you walk closer and repeat the instruction. She still does not respond, and you ask a third time. She ignores the question again, so you choose a book and begin to read. Gabriella listens to the first few pages but then walks away.
Social	Casey is learning to interact with his peers, and you are facilitating play between Casey and a friend. Casey is building a tower with blocks. When he reaches for the next block, you ask David to hand him a block. Casey takes the block from David and adds it to the tower. You then get his attention and say to him, "Casey, give a block to David."	Casey ignores this instruction and goes to put another block on top of the tower. You quickly put your hand on top of the tower to prevent this action, and point to David while repeating your instruction. Casey hands the block to David, who puts it on top of the tower.	Casey ignores this instruction and puts another block on top of the tower. You repeat the instruction a second time, but Casey knocks over the tower of blocks instead. David becomes bored and leaves the interaction.

COMPONENT 2: CLEAR AND APPROPRIATE INSTRUCTION

A clear and appropriate instruction is easy for the student to understand and is at, or just above, the student's developmental level.

Identifying a clear and appropriate instruction requires knowledge of a student's abilities. What is understandable for one student may be too advanced for another. You should know the language, play, and social abilities of each student; her overall ability to attend; whether she has learned the skill being presented; and even how she is performing the day the instruction is provided.

Uninterrupted Instructions

Clear instructions must be uninterrupted. That is, if you provide an instruction to a student, not only should your student be paying attention to the interaction, but you should too. It is important to give an instruction at a time when you can observe the student's response and assist with feedback. In a group setting, this may mean asking a question of the entire group (e.g., "What day is it today?") and responding to the student or students who answer appropriately. There will be times when another student needs immediate attention or other emergencies occur; however, ideally, attention should be provided to the student or group until a response has been made.

It is better not to provide an instruction at all than to fail to follow through.

Clear and Appropriate Language Expectations

Students with autism may vary greatly in both the type of language responses they provide and the level of language they under-

stand. Some students may have difficulty speaking, but can communicate using other methods (such as picture communication, sign language, or gesture). As a general rule, if a student is verbal, try to use language that is just above the student's expressive language ability (e.g., one level more complex than a student produces). A student who does not have good receptive language cannot be expected to respond to a command with two or three steps, such as "Pick up the pens and put them in your desk." This student may require you to model putting pens in the desk, or to use a more simple instruction such as "Pens in." Use each student's current language and skill level to help you determine what clear instructions for each student might be. For example, if a student has a goal of responding to one-step directions, then two- or three-step directions are too difficult. If a student is learning to use single words, then your instructions and prompts should be one to three words in length. A hierarchy of communication skills, listed in the order in which they are usually mastered by typically developing children, is provided in *Table 3.3*.

 Further information on play skill development can be found at *www.alf.dk/data/images/generalforsamling%202009/wordplayho.doc*

Clear and Appropriate Play Expectations

Students with autism also demonstrate great variability in play skills. Research indicates that the developmental appropriateness of cues is related to acquisition of new play skills. For example, one study found that when new play skills were being taught to students with autism, developmentally appropriate play skills tended to be acquired quickly, to occur spontane-

TABLE 3.3. Developmental Progression of Skills

Use this table to help determine the appropriate level of cue for each student.

Skill type	Skill level	Sample instructions at developmental level	Sample instructions above developmental level
Receptive communication	Gestural	Hold up a bucket and point inside.	Say, "Roll," or "In." Gesture may be needed to assist in responding.
	Single words	Say, "Ball," paired with open-hand prompt.	"Roll the ball," or "Block goes in."
	Phrase speech	"Sit in the chair."	"Push the green ball."
	Reciprocal communication	"Time to sit at your desk."	"Get the puzzle and give it to Joe."
Expressive communication	Preverbal	Hold up ball and model pointing to it.	Hold up ball and model saying, "Ball."
	Single words	Hold up ball and wait expectantly.	Hold up ball and model saying, "Throw the ball."
	Phrase speech	Hold up ball and model saying, "Roll the ball."	Hold up ball and say, "What do you want?" or "I have a ball."
	Reciprocal communication	Hold up the ball and say, "This red ball rolls fast!"	Hold up a ball and prompt, "I'm going to toss the ball in the bucket."
Play skills	Sensory–motor	Model feeling or squishing play clay.	Model stacking rings on a peg.
	Functional play	Model putting balls in tube or completing a puzzle; provide verbal instructions.	Model feeding a doll; say, "Feed the baby."
	Early pretend play (single-step actions)	Model talking on a toy phone; say, "Talk to Mommy."	Model pouring juice from an empty pitcher and say, "Baby wants juice too."
	Multiple pretend play actions	Model feeding self, doll, and peer, then driving the car to the store to get more snacks.	Provide blanket, plates, and cups and say, "Let's have a picnic!"
	Reciprocal play	Provide costumes for role playing with peers and say, "Let's play superheroes!"	Provide board games for two players that involve turn taking during free-play time.

ously, and to generalize to new toys. In contrast, children did not acquire play skills that were too advanced for them. Assessing a student's current level of play is therefore important for identifying which new skills should be taught. A clear and appropriate instruction for your student would be at, or just above, the level of play that the student can produce on her own. For example, for a student who has never played by putting his cars into a toy garage, a situational placement of a car and toy garage in the play area would not be considered a clear opportunity to respond. This student may need direct instruction and modeling, such as "Put the car in the garage," to respond to the opportunity. After the student has learned to complete the task with the direct instruction, a situational placement may be very clear for the student and encourage initiation and spontaneous play. A hierarchy of play skills, listed in the order in which they are usually mastered by typically developing children, is also provided in *Table 3.3*. You can complete a brief assessment of your student's play skills using *Handout 2: Object Play Level Progression*, found in *Part IV*.

"It's fun to have fun but you have to know how."—The Cat in the Hat *by Dr. Seuss*

Many children with autism do not learn to play with objects in the same way as their peers do. Teaching specific play skills increases the repertoire of activities a student can use for fun, spontaneous play. Eventually, play skills acquired through CPRT will be used independently by the student.

Increasing Expectations

As your student learns new skills and meets individualized learning goals, the types of language and social cues she understands will change. Early in each student's development, instructions will probably need to be very short, direct, and specific to the exact response you are teaching. As a student begins to understand language and social interaction, your instructions can include longer phrases and sentences, directions with more than one step, and perhaps even comments. It is important to be familiar with each student's language comprehension ability in order to provide instructions that she can understand. Remember that all instructions should be provided when the student is motivated and paying attention (see *Component 1*). It is also important to mix up more difficult instructions with simpler ones to keep motivation high (see *Component 3*).

Statement or Question Format

It is natural and important to include both statements and questions when you communicate with your students. However, you should be intentional about the specific words and tone of voice associated with both forms of communication. Sometimes adults use language and intonation associated with questioning when they are actually asking a student to follow an instruction or to repeat a verbal model. For example, you should usually state, "Time to clean up," instead of asking, "Are you ready to clean up?" You are teaching your student to answer questions as well as follow instructions, so if you ask an "Are you ready ... " question, you need to be prepared for the answer—which may be "No!" In addition, if you want your student to repeat the word "car" after you ask, "What do you want?", be sure you model the word in a statement intonation; otherwise, your student may learn to use inappropriate vocal intonation when answering questions.

If you are providing an instruction that you would like the student to complete, make it a statement, not a question.

COMPONENT 3: EASY AND DIFFICULT TASKS (MAINTENANCE/ACQUISITION)

Provide a mixture of easy and difficult tasks to increase motivation.

CPRT involves using both easy and difficult tasks, rather than continuously increasing task difficulty. Tasks that the student has mastered and can complete consistently and easily are called **maintenance tasks**. Tasks that are new, or continue to be difficult for the student, are called **acquisition tasks**. Use a mixture of tasks, requiring students to play, communicate, and perform both at levels that are easier for them (maintenance) and at more advanced levels (acquisition). Although there is no set rule, try to use maintenance tasks approximately 50% of the time. This can be altered, depending on the student (a highly motivated student may benefit from more acquisition tasks, and a tired or frustrated student may need more maintenance tasks) or the environment (a student may need a simpler instruction when there are many possible distractions in the classroom). This mixture of task difficulties is important for several reasons:

- *It increases motivation.* Putting in some easy tasks maintains the student's experience of success, while still allowing you to help move him forward in learning new skills.

- *It is developmentally appropriate.* Using skills of varying developmental levels is consistent with the behavior of typically developing children, who use a mixture of play and language levels. For example, once a student learns to pretend, she does not stop playing with puzzles. Similarly, just because a student has learned to speak in full sentences, such as "May I have a cookie, please?", this does not stop him from responding more succinctly, "I wanna cookie." It is thus natural and appropriate for students with autism to act and respond at varying levels.

- *It increases spontaneity.* One of the most difficult aspects of teaching a student with autism is dependence on prompts or lack of spontaneous responding. Interspersing maintenance and acquisition skills can

help to encourage spontaneity. Teaching new, difficult skills requires more support, or prompting. However, by interspersing easier tasks, you provide the student with an opportunity to spontaneously request, play, or follow a simple instruction without your help. This will increase both confidence and natural use of skills. This may be one of the most important reasons for rewarding students for the spontaneous use of simple language and play, even when you know they can do better with your help.

In *Table 3.4*, several scenarios are provided in which the teacher is providing a student with an opportunity to respond. Notice the likely difference in student response if the opportunities provided are a mix of easy and difficult tasks versus all difficult tasks.

COMPONENT 4: SHARED CONTROL (STUDENT CHOICE/TURN TAKING)

Share control by following your student's lead, providing choices of activities and materials, and taking turns with your student.

Controlling the learning environment includes choosing the materials, location, and goals for learning. Typically, a teacher maintains full control of the learning environment. However, in CPRT, sharing control of the learning environment with your student is another tool to increase motivation. Generally, people are more motivated or interested in learning if they get to choose the topic or activity. For example, if you like to take pictures, you are more likely to read a book on photography than a book that describes great football quarterbacks. If you find a physical activity you enjoy, like hiking in the woods, you are more likely to exercise. In the same way, students with autism will be more motivated to interact

TABLE 3.4. Easy and Difficult Tasks: Examples

This table provides examples of how to mix easy and difficult tasks.

Type	Setting	Easy and difficult tasks	Only difficult tasks
Language	Hans is playing with a ball drop and is learning to combine words. You join him in the play area and take each ball when it comes down the chute. You hold up a ball and model the phrase "Red ball" for Hans to repeat. He does so, and you give him the ball. He then points to another ball in your hand and says, "Green!"	You hand Hans the green ball to reward his spontaneous single word. You hold up the next ball and say, "Orange." Hans responds by saying, "Orange." You give him the orange ball, and he puts it down the chute. At the next opportunity, you help Hans repeat the two-word phrase "Orange ball," before giving him access to the ball.	Because you want Hans to use two words, you respond by modeling saying, "Green ball." Hans says, "Green!" and you again model saying, "Green ball." This occurs several times. Hans gets frustrated and walks away from the ball drop.
Academic	You give each student a list of topics (e.g., popular movies, outdoor activities, and holidays) to write about in their daily journal. Kara is learning to write five-sentence paragraphs with a topic sentence and conclusion.	On Kara's list of topics, you write "Paragraph" next to some topics and "Three sentences" next to others. This helps Kara to remain motivated to complete the entire list, and it helps her maintain practiced skills as well as work on new ones.	You tell Kara she needs to write five-sentence paragraphs for all the topics on the list. She writes paragraphs for the first two topics, but then becomes distracted and starts doodling on her paper.
Play	Steven is playing with an elephant figurine and a circus play set. He is just starting to sequence pretend play actions, such as giving a figurine a bath and putting it to sleep. You grab a monkey figurine and join Steven in the play area.	You model swinging the monkey on the trapeze and tell Steven, "Swing the elephant," which he does successfully. Next Steven pretends to feed the elephant, and you do the same with the monkey. You then tell Steven, "Give the elephant a bath and then put him to sleep," which he does.	You tell Steven, "Swing the elephant and give him a kiss," which he does successfully. Next you say, "Run really fast and then feed the elephant. He's hungry!" Steven makes the elephant run in a circle, but then loses interest and begins picking at the trunk.

when they are engaged with toys, activities, or conversation topics they enjoy. Many students with autism have difficulty attending to their teacher and peers because they lack motivation for social interaction. By incorporating a student's interests into a task or interaction, you increase the likelihood that the student will be motivated to attend. Because attention is critical for learning, sharing control can increase the overall number of goals your student achieves. However, it is also important to remember

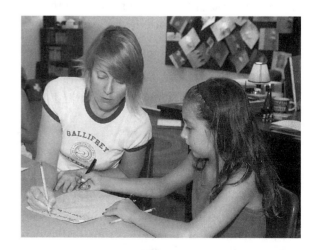

that this component emphasizes *shared* control, so it remains important for you to have control of materials, a clear understanding of the goals of the activity, and ultimate responsibility for the learning interaction. There are several methods you can use to share control with your student.

Incorporate Your Student's Preferred Materials

When you are preparing to teach a new skill, gather materials that are conducive to teaching this skill. For example, if you are introducing number identification, you may have flash cards, worksheets, or a video that presents the numbers 1 through 10. When sharing control with a student, you should be intentional about finding materials that the student enjoys and that can be used to teach the specific skill. For example, when you are teaching number identification, if a student enjoys puzzles, use a puzzle with numbers; if a student enjoys scribbling with crayons, use crayons and paper to write out the numbers; if a student is highly motivated for computer time, use the computer to type out each number in a large font.

The key to shared control is to provide the student with an opportunity to choose at least a portion of each activity.

When teaching very young students, or those with significant delays, you may have to observe them and infer their preferences or conduct a preference assessment. However, if your students can make choices, present one, such as "Computer or coloring?" You thus determine the goal of instruction, but your student shares control by choosing the materials or specific activity used to address that goal.

Follow Your Student's Lead

Allow the student to help determine when to move from one activity to the next. If your student initially selects coloring, continue coloring until she chooses to move on to something else. This creates an opportunity for the student to communicate that she's "all done," or to ask for the new activity, and it maximizes her motivation. Whenever possible, comply with the student's requests, in order to help her learn that appropriate communication results in desirable changes in the environment. This will also increase motivation. However, students with autism can often have difficulty with changing tasks too quickly or staying with one task for extended periods of time.

Incorporate Turn Taking

Turn taking is another way you can share control with a student. Turn taking involves a give-and-take interaction between the student and another peer or adult. Thus, if your student chooses to play with a car, you can take turns rolling, describing, and racing the car with him. Turn taking allows you to provide appropriate language and play models, demonstrate the give-and-take of social interaction, and regain control of teaching materials. Turns can be very brief if a student has difficulty paying attention while someone else has control of the materials. However, acting silly and incorporating the student into your turn may help maintain the student's attention when you are taking a turn. When you are working with a small group of students, it may be helpful to try turn taking during routine activities, such as circle or snack time. During snack time, turn taking may involve waiting for a peer to offer more pretzels or other snack foods. If the students know what is expected and can easily participate in an activity, it is often easier to keep their attention.

Turn taking is a component that's easy to forget. Be sure to model appropriate behaviors during your turn.

Maintain Safety and Appropriateness

It is important, and probably somewhat of a relief, to know that a student should not have total control. The student should not be allowed to engage in dangerous (e.g., aggressive, self-injurious) or inappropriate behavior. In these circumstances, you must assume control. Sometimes there is a fine line between appropriate and inappropriate opportunities for instruction. For example, stereotypic or self-stimulatory behavior may be highly motivating for a student, and can therefore be an excellent teaching tool. A student who loves to jump could be instructed to "Count to 7" with seven accompanying jumps. In contrast, it is probably inappropriate for a student who enjoys flipping the light switch to use this activity to practice counting, as it will disrupt the rest of the class.

In *Table 3.5*, several scenarios are provided in which the teacher is providing a student with an opportunity to respond. Notice the likely difference in student response if the teacher is sharing control with the student versus if the teacher is being directive and not allowing any student input.

COMPONENT 5: MULTIPLE CUES (BROADENING ATTENTION)

Use multiple examples of materials and concepts to ensure broad understanding.

Every time a new skill is learned, it involves associating **multiple cues**. A cue is a feature of an object or situation that you use to gather information and respond appropriately. You learn to link the spoken word "car" to a car as a physical object, based on multiple cues of a four-wheeled vehicle carrying passengers (i.e., shape, sound, function). If you were to say the word "car" in response to seeing a bicycle, it would mean that you do not know the cues related to "car." Similarly, you learn that the combination of waving and saying "good-bye" indicates someone is leaving. When you meet someone for the first time, you hear his name; feel the firmness of his handshake; and observe his hair color, eyeglasses, and style of dress. All of these cues provide critical information about this new acquaintance and help you identify this person the next time you meet.

Learning occurs when you understand the association between two or more features of a situation in your environment.

Since learning requires associating particular response behaviors with related cues (or antecedents), it is important that a student be able to attend to multiple cues in the environment. Although such learning is not a problem for typically developing children, children with autism can have difficulty learning when attention to simultaneous multiple cues is required. The tendency to attend to only one component of a complex cue is called **stimulus overselectivity**. Perhaps you can recall instances where a student has demonstrated this attentional deficit. Here are some examples from our own experience:

- A child only recognized his father when the father was wearing his glasses. When the father removed his glasses, the child responded as if the father were a stranger. It was apparent that the child had only attended to the glasses when learning who "Dad" was.

TABLE 3.5. Shared Control: Examples

This table illustrates varying outcomes of lessons using varying levels of shared control.

Type	Setting	Sharing control	Not sharing control
Play	You are working on an insect puzzle with Jerome, who loves bugs. He is learning to complete a puzzle independently, but he prefers to stack the pieces. You take all the puzzle pieces at the start of the activity.	You hold up two pieces of the puzzle, and Jerome points to one. You give him the piece. You then say, "Buzz, buzz, buzz—bug!" and place the next piece in the puzzle yourself as a model. You encourage Jerome to place his piece in the puzzle. When he is successful, you allow him to stack two pieces. This alternating pattern continues as Jerome completes the puzzle.	You require Jerome to put each piece in the puzzle to gain access to more pieces. He tries to stack the pieces and doesn't understand the task. He becomes frustrated and throws the puzzle.
Academic	Your students are completing a math activity at their desks. Susie is learning to complete simple multiplication problems.	You offer Susie a choice of pencils ("Would you like a heart pencil or a green pencil?") and let her choose which problem to do first. Every few problems, you model a solution and allow Susie to write it down on her paper. Susie completes all the problems.	You give Susie a heart pencil because you know she likes hearts. You point to the first problem and tell Susie, "Start here." Susie does several problems and you tell her, "Good job!" after each one, but she soon works more slowly and requires redirection.
Language	You are having snack with your students, and you are serving several types of fruit. You offer the tray of fruit to each student and require them to communicate to receive their desired snack.	You offer the tray to Kelly and ask, "What do you want to eat?" She responds, "Eat apple." You then offer the tray to Ryan and ask, "Grapes or pear?" He responds, "Pear." Next, you tell your students, "I will eat an apple—yum!" and take a slice of apple for yourself. You then continue offering fruit to the rest of the students in the circle.	You offer apples to all the students and have them respond according to their language level.

- A little girl worked with her teacher for over 6 months and knew the teacher's name. The teacher had long hair, but one day she decided to cut it short. The next day in class, the little girl walked up to the teacher and asked, "What's your name?" She had no idea who the teacher was. The child had learned to identify the teacher on the basis of her hair, and when that was changed, the child could no longer identify her.

- A mother reported that every time she wore new shoes, her son with autism became upset and confused.

All of these examples are instances where a child had attended to only one (and often an irrelevant) cue when learning. The children in these examples failed to pay attention to the many, more permanent cues (facial features, body type, height, etc.) that allow most of us to recognize others even when some details of their appearance change.

For many children with autism, early intervention and the use of varied instructions, materials, and examples can increase appropriate attention and responding. Therefore, it is important to use different materials and methods to teach the same concept. That is why lessons should be taught in various settings, during different activities. For example, when you are teaching a student to add, if only specific blocks are used to teach the concept, the student may think that addition is only done with those blocks and may not understand the broader concept of addition of any items. Using blocks, pens, jacks, and balls to teach addition can help broaden the student's idea of what addition means. The same is true when you are teaching new words, phrases, and play activities. For most of your students, this type of teaching will be sufficient to provide attention to simultaneous multiple cues, because they have learned that they need to do this in order to understand the lesson and respond appropriately.

However, some children with autism have more severe difficulties with overselectivity. These students may need more structured tasks to learn to expand their attention to multiple cues at the same time. Repeated practice with tasks that require response to multiple cues can help the student attend to multiple cues simultaneously in new tasks. For these students with autism, practice in using multiple cues can lead to a general broadening (or normalizing) of attention. To teach these skills, you can present cues for which the correct response requires responding to multiple cues, such as shape and size, or color and texture. Such tasks are called **conditional discriminations**.

To illustrate, a student who is asked to get her brown jacket will have to attend to both color and object in order to respond

correctly. This is because she probably has many items of clothing, and many of them may be brown. Another student has chosen to play with a set of colored blocks of different shapes, and there are circles, squares, and other shapes in the different colors. You can use conditional discriminations to ensure that the student learns both color *and* shape by holding all the blocks in a bucket and having the student ask for blocks by labeling both the color and shape (e.g., "I need a red square," or "Please give me a green circle"). In order to receive a block, the student needs to attend to and label both shape and color. It can be challenging to think of materials that naturally lend themselves to instructions and opportunities to respond involving conditional discriminations. *Table 3.6* provides several ideas with materials that are probably already available in your classroom.

In *Table 3.7*, several scenarios are provided in which the teacher is providing a student with an opportunity to respond. These examples allow you to compare situations in which the teacher involves response to multiple cues versus only single cues.

Important caveat: Typically developing children do not reliably respond to simultaneous multiple cues until approximately 36 months of age.

Keep in mind that it is not appropriate to use multiple cues to teach children with autism who have a developmental age of less than 36 months. Many children with autism enter special education classrooms at 36 months of age chronologically, but at a lower developmental level or mental age. The best way to use CPRT to address the needs of these students, therefore, is to focus on the other elements of the protocol and not use multiple cues.

TABLE 3.6. Examples of Materials for Teaching Multiple Cues

Many materials already in your classroom can be used to teach conditional discriminations to students with autism who are overselective.

Material type	Suggested pairs of features	Examples of materials
Vehicles	Type and size, type and color	Small, medium, and large examples of buses, cars, and trucks in different colors
Books	Subject and size, color and size	Large and small books of different subjects and colors
Writing utensils	Type and color	Pens, pencils, crayons, and markers in different colors
Dolls/character figurines	Size and identity	Large and small dolls of several of the student's favorite characters
Animal figurines	Type and family member	Mommy and baby animals of several types
Blocks	Quantity and color, size and color, shape and color	Various shapes of blocks in several colors and/or sizes
Snacks	Texture and quantity, color and type	Bite-sized snacks in several textures and/or colors

 For more information on overselectivity and how to use conditional discriminations to reduce overselectivity, take a look at the references under *Responding to Multiple Cues* in the *Suggested Readings* list at the end of the book.

Watch What Happens: Student Behavior

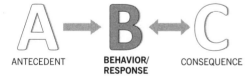

ANTECEDENT   BEHAVIOR/RESPONSE   CONSEQUENCE

Once you have presented an opportunity to respond, the next step is to observe your student's behavior in response to that opportunity. How your student responds will determine what you do next, so it is important to watch closely. Observing your student will help you react to his behavior quickly and accurately. After observing your student's response, you must decide whether it is an appropriate or inappropriate reply to

the opportunity you have presented. Several factors, including environment, activity, student ability, and target skill, determine the appropriateness of your student's response. The different types of responses your student may give are discussed in more detail in the *Behavior* section of *Chapter 2*. *Table 3.8* provides a brief summary of the ways to classify your student's behavior in response to an opportunity.

 It is helpful to decide ahead of time what you will accept as a "reasonable attempt" from your student.

React: Consequence Strategies

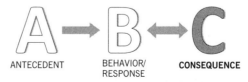

ANTECEDENT   BEHAVIOR/RESPONSE   **CONSEQUENCE**

As described in *Chapter 2*, consequences (the way you respond to student behavior)

TABLE 3.7. Multiple Cues: Examples

This table provides examples of teachers' incorporating responses to multiple cues versus a single cue in daily classroom activities.

Type	Setting	Multiple cues	Single cues
Play	Amir has chosen to play with a toy garage set. There are several vehicles of different types (e.g., trucks, buses, cars), and each of these vehicle types come in different colors.	While Amir moves the various vehicles around the garage, you take a turn, commenting, "I'm driving the red bus." You block access to the garage with a green car and give Amir an expectant look. He says, "Move car!" You respond by saying, "Which one?" Amir replies, "Move green car!" and you move the car so he can drive his chosen vehicle into the garage.	While Amir moves the various vehicles around the garage, you take a turn with a bus and then block access to the garage with your hand. Amir says, "Move hand!" and you move your hand away so he can drive his chosen vehicle into the garage.
Academic	Carolyn has requested to play with marbles and drop them into a box. You ensure that the marble set contains marbles of different sizes and colors. You also decide that this is a good opportunity to teach Carolyn number concepts.	You ask Carolyn to drop five small green marbles into the box.	You ask Carolyn to drop five marbles into the box.
Language	Dennis loves to play with puzzles and has chosen a puzzle with mother and baby animals. The puzzle pieces are animals of different sizes (e.g., mother giraffe and baby giraffe, mother elephant and baby elephant). You note that this is a good opportunity to help Dennis learn the prepositions *in* and *out*.	You take out the little elephant piece and say, "I'm taking the baby elephant *out*." You then suggest that Dennis take the mother giraffe "*out*." This type of interaction continues, with various-sized animals being taken in and out.	You take out the baby tiger and say, "I'm taking out the tiger." You then suggest that Dennis take out an elephant.

TABLE 3.8. Types of Behavioral Responses

This table illustrates the various responses a student may make to your opportunity to respond.

Response	Description
Appropriate response	Falls within the range of skills you are targeting.
Reasonable attempt	Serves the same function as the target skill, without the same accuracy or complexity.
Inappropriate response	Unrelated to the interaction or disruptive; failure to respond.
Incorrect response	Incorrect.

are the means you have to teach new skills, maintain skills, and decrease unwanted behaviors. Consequences are what happen right after a behavior occurs, and the nature and timing of these consequent events determine how behavior will be affected. Just as important as the types of consequences is the manner in which they are presented. Please refer to the *Consequences* section of *Chapter 2* for a review of the types of consequences. *Table 3.9* provides a brief summary of the ways in which you may respond to your student's behavior. CPRT Components 6, 7, and 8 involve the effective delivery of consequences.

COMPONENT 6: DIRECT REINFORCEMENT

Provide reinforcement that is naturally or directly related to the activity or behavior.

Direct reinforcement is directly related to the preceding behavior. For example, if a student says the word "Car" when motivated to play with a toy car, then access to the toy car is a direct reinforcer. Access to the car is directly related to the student's saying the word. In contrast, **indirect reinforcement** occurs when the response and the consequence are unrelated. If a teacher holds up a picture of a car and asks, "What is it?" the student says, "Car," and the teacher says, "Good talking!" or gives the student a cookie, the consequence is not directly related to the response.

Generalization (using a behavior in other environments or with other materials) and **maintenance** of acquired behavior are both greatly enhanced when direct reinforcement is used. Consider how direct reinforcement relates to language learning in our natural environment. Going to a fast-food restaurant and saying, "Hamburger, please," results in getting a hamburger. You would be disappointed to instead hear, "Good talking!" A hamburger is direct reinforcement in this case because it is directly related to what you said. "Good talking!" is not direct reinforcement because it is not directly related to what you said. (That is, at a fast-food restaurant, if you say, "Hamburger, please," you can be pretty certain you will get the food rather than praise for talking.) The problem with using indirect consequences is that the real-world environment does not supply them. Thus newly acquired skills are not reinforced or maintained in the environment. A student who expects to receive a piece of candy or a gold star for talking will be unlikely to use speech in the natural environment, where candy and gold stars are typically not given for talking.

TABLE 3.9. Types of Consequences

This table illustrates the types of consequences you may provide to your student following his behavioral response.

Consequence	Description
Positive reinforcement	Presentation of a desired item after a behavior, which leads to an increase in the behavior.
Negative reinforcement	Removal of an undesirable situation after a behavior, which leads to an increase in the behavior.
Punishment	Presentation of an undesirable situation of item after a behavior, which leads to a decrease in the behavior.
Extinction	Discontinuation of reinforcement, which leads to a decrease in the behavior.

Children acquire language because it is an effective way to change their environment, and the natural environment provides direct reinforcement.

It is important to point out that indirect reinforcers can be highly effective in teaching a new skill. However, the skill may only be demonstrated in the environment where it has been taught (i.e., where the indirect reinforcer is given). Since the natural environment does not provide these consequences, the behavior will probably be lost. A skill that has been taught with direct consequences will be under the control of natural consequences and should be maintained in the natural environment.

In *Table 3.10*, several scenarios are provided in which the teacher needs to provide a consequence for a particular student behavior. Notice the difference between the reinforcement directly related to the activity and that which is indirectly related.

COMPONENT 7:
CONTINGENT CONSEQUENCE
(IMMEDIATE AND APPROPRIATE)

Present consequences immediately, based on the student's response.

Another important component of CPRT is that the consequence must be **contingent**—that is, dependent—upon the student's behavior. One aspect of contingency is that the consequence should be presented immediately after a behavior occurs. In fact, the strength and effectiveness of a consequence are directly related to its timing. The more delayed the consequence is after a response, the weaker its effect. Because the immediacy of the consequence is so important, note that the behavior occurring just before the consequence is the behavior most affected by it.

The sooner the consequence is delivered after a response, the stronger its effect.

Consequences are not always immediate. However, most of us can use language to make the consequence more contingent by saying something like "You did a great job in class today," or "Thank you for taking out the trash last night." Unfortunately, many of the students with autism in your class may not have sufficient language to mediate consequences across time, so the immediacy of the consequence is particularly important. For example, imagine that a teacher notices a student misbehaving on the other side of the room. By the time she can navigate across the room to provide a consequence ("William, stop that"), several seconds have elapsed. Just when she gets over to him, he is being quiet. By presenting the consequence at this time, she is inadvertently punishing William for being quiet (what he was doing just before the consequence) and thus discouraging this behavior. In this situation, the teacher should instead redirect William's behavior to an appropriate activity once she reaches him, and utilize an immediate consequence for misbehaving at the next available opportunity.

Contingency also means that the consequence must be dependent upon the student's response, in the sense that the consequence would not be presented if there were no behavior. A reinforcer that is presented randomly (i.e., not dependent upon a behavior) is ineffective at changing behavior. Randomly winning the lottery will not make someone more productive or hard-working, but a bonus for a job well done will increase productivity. In the same way, saying, "Good talking!" to a student at random intervals will not increase the likelihood that the student will speak, but responding to a student's language in meaningful ways will increase speech.

TABLE 3.10. Direct Reinforcement: Examples

The examples in this table illustrate the difference between providing direct and indirect rewards to your student.

Type	Setting	Direct	Indirect
Language	You are teaching Raquel to identify actions. You show her a picture of a child jumping and ask, "What is he doing?"	Raquel responds, "Jumping," and is allowed to bounce on a trampoline for several seconds.	Raquel responds, "Jumping." You tell her, "Great job, that's jumping!" and hand her a cookie.
Social	You are teaching Johnny to approach a peer and ask a question. At recess, Johnny is interested in the swings. You facilitate Johnny in approaching Tom, who is playing on the swings.	You help Johnny ask Tom for a turn on the swing, and Tom gives him a turn. You push Johnny on the swing as a reward for successfully asking Tom a question.	You help Johnny ask Tom what his favorite color is. You push Johnny on the swing as a reward for successfully asking Tom a question.
Play	You are teaching Susie to engage in symbolic play. She has chosen a toy ranch set to play with, and you prompt her to pretend that a pencil is a fence.	Susie uses the pencil as a fence, and as a consequence you allow her to play with the ranch set as she pleases.	Susie uses the pencil as a fence, and as a consequence you let her choose the song for circle time.
Academic	You are teaching Carolyn to use prepositions. Carolyn has chosen to put together an animal puzzle. She chooses the rooster puzzle piece.	You put the rooster piece in a box and ask Carolyn, "Where is the rooster?" Carolyn replies, "In the box." You then give Carolyn the piece of the puzzle as a reward for answering the question correctly.	You take the puzzle pieces and tell Carolyn it's time to work. You show Carolyn a picture of a baby in a bathtub, and ask, "Where is the baby?" Carolyn replies, "In the bathtub." You then give Carolyn the rooster puzzle piece as a reward for answering the question correctly.

Like instructions, consequences must be clearly presented, so that the student can make a connection between the consequence and the behavior and can understand the nature of the consequence. To illustrate, imagine that you are trying to teach Shayla to draw a circle. After many, many attempts, Shayla is unable to draw the circle despite trying very hard. If you use a positive voice to say, "No, no, but I know you are trying, you cutie, you!", you are providing a confusing consequence. The content is both negative ("No, no") and positive ("you cutie, you!"). In addition, the tone is very positive. The student may misinterpret the consequence as positive reinforcement for the error.

A contingent consequence is one that is clear, depends on the occurrence of a behavior, and is presented as soon as possible following the behavior.

In *Table 3.11*, several scenarios are provided in which the teacher needs to provide a consequence for a particular student behavior. Notice the difference between the immediate, appropriate consequences

TABLE 3.11. Contingent Consequences: Examples

This table illustrates the difference between providing immediate, appropriate consequences and providing delayed, inappropriate consequences to your student.

Type	Setting	Contingent	Noncontingent
Language	You are reading a farm story with your class during circle time. You are asking each student to make the sound of an animal in the farm story. As Nurit makes a cow sound, you notice that Paul is also attempting to say, "Mooo." This is a relatively infrequent behavior for Paul, who is usually not communicative.	Immediately upon noticing Paul's behavior, you hand him a cow figurine. You then proceed around the circle, having the students name the animals.	You continue until you have finished having all the students in the circle name the animals. Then you turn to Paul and say, "I like the way you were saying, 'Mooo,' Paul." However, now Paul is silent.
Social	During a lesson with the whole class, Marta is being disruptive by wandering around the classroom and humming loudly instead of staying in her currently assigned work station.	As soon as Marta gets up and starts to wander, you say, "Marta, please be quiet and return to your seat." You then have a paraprofessional follow Marta back to her seat to ensure that she sits down.	When you see Marta get up and hum, you say, "Marta, what are you doing now?" and continue the lesson to the class. Marta stops humming but continues wandering around the classroom.
Academic	You are teaching Joey to identify shapes by placing them in a shape sorter. Upon hearing you say, "Circle," Joey puts the circle in the correct hole.	You exclaim, "Yes, that's a circle, Joey!" and allow him to line the remaining shapes up on the floor for a few seconds before holding up the next shape for him to put in.	You then say, "Now put in the square," which Joey does successfully. Next, you hand Susie a triangle and say, "Put in." Joey loses interest and walks away from the activity.

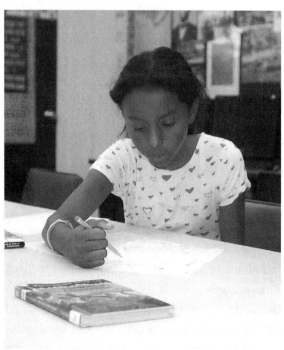

and the delayed, inappropriate (i.e., not dependent on the student's response) consequences.

COMPONENT 8:
REINFORCEMENT OF ATTEMPTS

Reward good trying to encourage your student to try again in the future.

The final CPRT component is reinforcement of attempts. As described in the *Behavior* section of *Chapter 2*, an **attempt** is a behavior that serves the same function as the target skill, without the accuracy or complexity of a "correct" response.

Provide reinforcement to the student for trying to answer correctly, even if the attempt is not his best response.

Reinforcing attempts can lead to increased responsivity. Suppose that a student is learning to label his favorite toy, a truck. He has said the word "truck" quite clearly on occasion, but on this particular trial the student only makes a "trrrr" sound instead of "truck," even after several prompts. The "trrr" response is a reasonable attempt at the word, so the student should be rewarded with the truck to reduce the possibility of frustration. Of course, the response has to be reasonable in the sense that it is close to what the student has shown he can do. If this student were to make a "bur" sound to request the truck, reinforcement should not be delivered, since "bur" is not advanced enough to indicate that the student is trying. Reinforce a broad range of responses, as opposed to only responses that are at least as good as those the student has performed before. By reinforcing attempts, you encourage more trying in the future.

Reinforcement of attempts is critical, because it increases student motivation. By reinforcing reasonable attempts at responding correctly and thus reinforcing a broader range of responses, you keep the amount of reinforcement high. When students with autism are reinforced for attempts, rather than for only correct responses, they are less frustrated and more motivated; are judged to be happier; and are less likely to engage in avoidance-motivated behaviors, such as crying, screaming, and trying to escape the teaching situation. In addition, reinforcement of attempts often leads to rapid progress on acquisition of new skills.

In *Table 3.12*, several scenarios are provided in which the teacher needs to provide a consequence for a particular student behavior. Notice the difference in the student's response to the teaching interaction when the student's good attempts are being reinforced versus when they are not.

Chapter Summary

CPRT has eight critical components. Five of these components are antecedent strategies, which are used to set up a naturalistic opportunity for students to respond. Antecedent strategies include (1) gaining the student's attention; (2) providing a clear and appropriate instruction or opportunity to respond; (3) mixing easy and difficult task expectations to increase motivation; (4) using shared control techniques, such as allowing student choice of materials or activities and peer or teacher turn taking to model behavior and gain control of the teaching materials; and (5) using multiple examples (varied materials and instructions) to help students learn to attend to multiple cues in their environment. Once the student produces a behavior, CPRT provides three consequence strategies to maximize learning through teacher feedback. These consequence strategies include (6) providing reinforcement that is directly related to the teaching activity; (7) providing contingent consequences that are immediate and based on the student's behavior; and (8) rewarding goal-directed attempts to ensure continued responding over time. These strategies, when used together, enhance motivation to learn, encourage the use of new skills in different settings, with varied materials and adults (generalization), and promote continued use of new skills over time (maintenance).

TABLE 3.12. Reinforcement of Attempts: Examples

This table illustrates teachers' rewarding students' good attempts at responding versus only accepting exactly correct responses or rewarding inadequate attempts.

Type	Setting	Attempt reinforced	Attempt not reinforced
Turn taking	Gina and Ken are learning to share. While Ken is quite verbal and can ask for a turn, Gina is just learning. While playing with a Mr. Potato Head, Ken takes a turn and puts on the eyes. Gina picks up the mouth to put on the toy. You prompt Gina to say, "Turn," and reach for the toy. Gina has never said, "Turn," but this time she says, "Tah."	You immediately help Ken give Gina the toy and praise her for good trying.	You prompt "Turn" again, because you are working on Gina's using the whole word. Gina repeats "Tah" and reaches for Mr. Potato Head. You slowly repeat "Turn" a third time, and Gina becomes frustrated and throws the mouth at Ken.
Language	You are teaching Samir to ask for desired objects and activities by combining a verb with a noun. You see Samir reaching for a drum and prompt him to say, "Play drum." Samir says, "Pluh." You have heard Samir say the words "play" and "drum" very clearly many times in the past.	You wait for Samir to give a more correct response, because he is highly motivated for the drum. Samir does not, so you again prompt, "Play drum." Now Samir says, "Pluh druh," and you give him the drum as a reward for his good trying.	You give Samir the drum immediately, without waiting for a more correct response. Samir will probably not be motivated to give his best response next time. (Notice that different responses are expected for Gina and Samir, because they are at different levels.)
Play	Heather likes to play with the ring stacker, but she has trouble putting the rings on the peg. She prefers to spin the rings rather than stack them. After Heather picks up the red ring, you say, "Put red ring on." Heather starts to spin the ring, and you gently interfere with the spinning and move Heather's hand toward the peg. Heather stops spinning the ring and holds it close to the peg.	You help Heather complete the remainder of the action and put the ring on the peg while saying, "Wow, you put it on!" and allow her to spin the ring briefly as a reward for putting the ring on. Heather picks up the next ring and holds it close to the peg.	You tell her, "No, put it on the ring," and put the ring back on the floor for Heather to try again. Heather picks up the ring, starts spinning it again, and resists all further prompts.

PART II

Next Steps with CPRT

CHAPTER 4
Group Instruction with CPRT

CHAPTER OVERVIEW

The original PRT protocol was developed for use with students in one-on-one settings. However, the CPRT components have been adapted for use in either individual or group settings. This chapter is designed to help you use CPRT in a variety of lessons throughout the day. Researchers have learned how to implement CPRT in group settings by collaborating with teachers to adapt the procedures. This section provides examples of activities that allow you to use CPRT components in two different situations. For each component, examples are provided for individual students within a group activity, and then examples and tips are given for activities in which the entire group must work together.

The following sections are included:

Component 1: Student Attention
    Targeting Individuals within a Group
    Group Instruction

Component 2: Clear and Appropriate Instruction
    Targeting Individuals within a Group
    Group Instruction

Component 3: Easy and Difficult Tasks (Maintenance/Acquisition)
    Targeting Individuals within a Group
    Group Instruction

Component 4: Shared Control (Student Choice/Turn Taking)
    Targeting Individuals within a Group
    Group Instruction

Component 5: Multiple Cues (Broadening Attention)
    Targeting Individuals within a Group
    Group Instruction

Component 6: Direct Reinforcement
    Targeting Individuals within a Group
    Group Instruction

Component 7: Contingent Consequence (Immediate and Appropriate)
    Targeting Individuals within a Group
    Group Instruction

Component 8: Reinforcement of Attempts
    Targeting Individuals within a Group
    Group Instruction

This chapter has a corresponding training lecture on the DVD accompanying this manual (*CPRT Session 3: CPRT with Groups and for Student Goals*).

Once you have mastered using CPRT with individual students, you are ready to begin using the same approach with a group of students. Though it can be challenging at first to incorporate all the components of CPRT and manage students in a group simultaneously, practicing these skills over time in a variety of activities will help strengthen your ability to use CPRT. It may be helpful to start by using CPRT in a group in a single, daily activity that is highly motivating to your students. This will allow you to refine your skills with repeated practice in the same setting. No matter how you begin, you will see that CPRT is a valuable approach for addressing student goals during group activities.

COMPONENT 1: STUDENT ATTENTION

Be sure your students are paying attention before you ask them to do or say something.

Ensuring attention from a group of students can be more difficult than keeping one student's attention. However, the same methods for gaining attention that are described in *Chapter 3* can often be used when working with a group.

 Be sure you fully understand and feel comfortable implementing CPRT with individual students before beginning to implement CPRT in a group (see *Chapter 3*).

Targeting Individuals within a Group

Choose Motivating Activities

When you are working with a group, it is still important to use toys, topics, and activities that your students enjoy. When you are working in a small group and asking students to respond individually, you may be able to individualize the activity to increase student motivation. For example, during a calendar activity, each student may have an opportunity to come to the front to respond about the day, date, weather, and so on. If Samantha enjoys numbers, having her identify the date and place the number on the calendar may increase her motivation to pay attention during circle time. Allowing other students to go first and providing Samantha a turn contingent upon good attention may further increase her ability to attend to the entire activity. Similarly, a group of students may be working on handwriting around a small table. Writing letters or words related to favorite cartoon pictures may increase motivation for this activity. An obstacle course designed for work on large motor tasks may permit jumping on a trampoline for one student and climbing over a bolster for another.

Be Close

Proximity is still important in a group situation. When asking each student to respond, ensure that you are near the student, and make it clear that a response is expected.

Be Fun and Engaging

The more you enjoy yourself, the more your students will enjoy playing with you and listening to you. You can vary your volume and animation for each student as you require a response. Be silly or incorporate surprises, and encourage students to have fun with their responses, in order to keep the other students watching and learning throughout the activity.

Keep It Natural

Use a natural tone of voice with the group, and avoid repeatedly calling students' names or asking for attention.

Build Tolerance for Attention to the Teaching Activity

To reduce frustration for both you and your students, begin by expecting only brief periods of attention during group activities. Every student does not need to remain with the group for the entire activity. Perhaps one of the students has difficulty paying attention when he is not directly required to respond. Escort him back to the table for his turn, and allow him to ask to leave the table when his turn is complete. Then increase the amount of time he remains with the group as he is able to pay attention

for longer periods of time. Just as with the individual activities, your expectations can increase as your students can pay attention for longer periods of time.

Group Instruction

Choose Motivating Activities

Choosing motivating activities can be more challenging in a large group, because the activity needs to be motivating for all of the students involved. Allowing turn taking and providing manipulatives can help keep children engaged. For example, reading a book while students choose items that represent characters from the book, or having students act out scenes from the story, can be very motivating. An obstacle course designed for work on large motor tasks may include a trampoline at the end to encourage the children to complete the other tasks. Observe your class members and the types of things they like, and try to incorporate these things into lessons that children may find difficult. Classroom themes may also be used to motivate students (see the *Using CPRT with School-Based Standards* section of *Chapter 6* for more information).

 Choosing materials that interest all the students in your group can maximize student attention. Compare preference assessments (see *Chapter 6*) among your students to find mutually motivating materials.

Be Close

When you are leading a large group, be in front of the students or have them situated so that they can all see you clearly. Place students with the most difficulty paying attention nearest to you or to a paraprofessional who can redirect their attention.

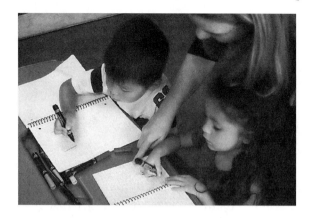

Be Fun and Engaging

Being fun and engaging can be especially important in a larger group to help keep all of the students' attention. Continue to be playful, silly, and creative, and watch your students' reactions to the things you do. Using movement, music, and high animation can keep the attention of the group. Remember to base your affect level on your students—some may need less animation to remain calm and engaged. Attempt to actively engage the students by encouraging them to repeat words, imitate hand movements, and hand materials to one another.

Structure the Environment

Using environmental supports can help keep the group engaged in a natural way. For example, carpet squares or chairs can help students understand where they should keep their bodies. You can also reduce distractions from hallways and other classroom spaces.

Build Tolerance for Attention to the Teaching Activity

Again, students may need to begin by spending short periods of time in larger-group activities. Large-group activities can be overwhelming for some students. It is important not to reinforce students for poor behavior by allowing them to leave a group activity

they do not enjoy. Instead, provide a way for a student who cannot remain attentive to ask to leave the activity, or allow the student to move away *before* the difficult behavior occurs. This will allow you to increase the time the student is expected to stay in the group, while keeping that student's attention and encouraging good behavior.

COMPONENT 2: CLEAR AND APPROPRIATE INSTRUCTION

A clear and appropriate instruction is easy for students to understand and is at, or just above, the students' developmental level.

Because what constitutes "clear and appropriate instruction" is different for each student, you may need to alter a cue or instruction to meet the needs of different students in the group (see *Component 2: Clear and Appropriate Instruction* in *Chapter 3* for a complete description of how to match instructions to each child's developmental level).

Targeting Individuals within a Group

Uninterrupted Instruction

When you are working with a group of students, interruption and distraction are much more likely to occur. Therefore, you need to pay particular attention to *following through* with each student. Several strategies may be useful in helping to ensure that instructions to individual students are not interrupted during group activities. One strategy is to use a pattern in the way instructions are provided, so that students can anticipate when it will be their turn. For example, if each student is asked to count a certain number of favorite objects by using the same rhythm, it will be easier for them to anticipate how and when they should respond. In addition, other students may be interested in observing and doing the same when it is their turn. Another strategy is to use an activity that engages each student for a few minutes while you move around the group. For example, have each student label colors and shapes, and then trace, draw, or color in a shape (depending upon the student's skill level) while you ask the same of the next student.

It is also important to guard against distractions you may experience. If you are focused on getting a response from Julianne, and Peter is fidgeting, it is best simply to focus on Julianne's response rather than interrupt your cue to reprimand Peter. This will help avoid repeated reprimands and instructions that cannot be backed up with a clear consequence. Peter can be rewarded for good attention and sitting still at other times during the activity. Of course, interruptions will occur. When this happens, simply provide the instruction or opportunity again when you can follow through.

Clear and Appropriate Expectations

Continue to use clear instructions for each student. At snack time, for example, some students can ask for a cracker using a complete sentence ("Sue, pass me the crackers"); others may use a sign or picture to ask for the crackers. When you are providing math instructions, one student may be asked simply to identify a number, while another must complete an addition problem.

Even when you are working in a group environment, instructions can be adapted to students' varying skill levels.

Similarly, when you are working on play skills, the same toy can be adapted for use at a variety of levels. For example,

when students are working with a train set, Donna might pretend to fix a broken wheel on the train, wash it, put it on the track, and drive a doll to the store. Once the train is at the store, Mikaela might be asked simply to drive the train back around the track without pretending. Jacqueline might drop the train cars into a box that Donna pretends is the garage. The students can learn to take turns as they model different levels of appropriate play for each other during the interaction.

 Refer to *Table 3.3* in *Chapter 3* for a hierarchy of language and play skills.

Group Instruction

Uninterrupted Instructions

When you are providing opportunities to a larger group of students, interruption and distraction may come from individual students within the group. You should be ready to give instructions before gaining the group's attention. That is, you don't want students to come to the activity and be required to wait a long time before the activity begins. If a particular student is disruptive, it may be beneficial to complete the interaction with the rest of the group, follow through with the appropriate reinforcement for the students who respond well, and then work individually with the disruptive student. If possible, ignore the disruptive student while you continue to work with the group, or ask a paraprofessional to assist you. This will serve to reduce the amount of attention the disruptive student receives for inappropriate behavior, ensure that instructions are not interrupted for the majority of the group, and reward the other students for appropriate behavior. If an interruption comes from outside the group (perhaps in the form of a phone call or a parent needing attention), complete the interaction before leaving the group whenever possible.

Clear and Appropriate Expectations

Even in a large-group environment, instructions can be adapted to varying skill levels. For example, perhaps you have asked the students to complete a writing assignment that involves writing a paragraph about their favorite movie. You may first provide the instruction verbally for those students with better language skills and require them to write a paragraph about the film. For other students, you may provide pictures of various movie examples known to be popular with the class, as well as a list of specific questions to answer about the movie. Other students may simply need to choose a picture of a favorite movie and copy the title of the film. During circle time, you may ask a question of the entire group (e.g., "What day is it today?") and respond to the student who answers appropriately, or to more than one student if needed. The next question may be simpler, targeting students who have more difficulty understanding language: "Today is ... " (while pointing to the word *Monday*).

It may be necessary to provide instructions in a variety of ways, such as using both auditory and visual cues when giving a group instruction.

Similarly, when you are working on play and social skills, the group activity can be adapted for use at a variety of levels. For example, if the class will be playing a game such as soccer, some students (those who understand the game well enough) may be assigned a specific position. Other students may need to play with a buddy, or may

be given a specific job, such as completing throw-ins or kicking the ball in a specific direction. Some students may be required to take turns with a toy, while others can learn to trade toys. Students may also use toys in a collaborative and cooperative manner, such as when one student "drives" a toy car to the gas station and another student "fills" the car with gas.

COMPONENT 3: EASY AND DIFFICULT TASKS (MAINTENANCE/ACQUISITION)

Provide a mixture of easy and difficult tasks to increase motivation.

Use both easy and difficult tasks rather than continuously increasing task difficulty, whether you are working individually or with a group.

Targeting Individuals within a Group

Component 3 can be used in a small group in basically the same way that it is used during individual sessions. Students should be provided both cues that are easy for them (maintenance tasks) and those that are more difficult (acquisition tasks). If a student has difficulty working in a group, an increase in maintenance tasks may be useful to maintain motivation. Group settings provide nice opportunities for students to model for each other, as what is difficult for one student may be easy for another. Students working at higher levels on particular tasks can serve as leaders for the group during work on that task. For example, at snack time, Betty may be required to ask the question "Mr. Snyder, may I have a cracker?" (acquisition task) for her first serving, and "More cracker, please" (maintenance task) for the second. Another student, Jillian, benefits from Betty's model. With Jillian, the teacher alternates between requiring "More cracker, please" (acquisition task) and "Cracker" (maintenance task) to request the snack.

Group Instruction

Maintenance and acquisition tasks are different for each student in the classroom, which makes using this strategy in a large group more challenging. However, instructions can be easier and harder for the group as a whole, increasing motivation and spontaneity for group activities. For example, if the group task is to play Simon Says, some instructions may involve language and others gestures or pictures. The group may be asked to complete a cooperative task, such as making something out of blocks, and you can include easier and more difficult structures for the students to build. This provides each student in the group with an opportunity to succeed, while still encouraging them to learn new skills. Students with more advanced skills can help students who need assistance, increasing everyone's social skills and feelings of competence.

COMPONENT 4: SHARED CONTROL (STUDENT CHOICE/TURN TAKING)

Share control by following your students' lead, providing choices of activities and materials, and taking turns with your students.

Maintaining shared control in the context of a group can be tricky. However, creative methods can be used to help students share control, thereby increasing their motivation to participate in group activities.

Maintain Safety and Appropriateness

Just as in the individual sessions, safety comes first. Additionally, the needs of the entire class must be considered when you are allowing students to make choices. This component of CPRT may not be appropriate for all group lessons or situations.

Targeting Individuals within a Group

Incorporate Your Student's Preferred Materials

Incorporating preferred materials can still be done relatively easily when you are targeting individuals within a group; however, it may take some preparation. At snack time, it may mean that several food and drink choices are available; during work on cutting skills, you may provide different pictures and shapes for students to cut out, based on each student's interests. At other times, students can choose specific items within the activity—for example, the color of pencil they would like to use, the type of objects they would like to count, the type of animal noise they would like to make, or the picture they would like to discuss. Remember, if a student perseverates on specific objects or materials, you can always encourage more complex behavior with those materials.

Incorporate preferred materials for each student in the group.

Follow Your Student's Lead

Allowing a student to help determine when to move from one activity to the next will also be more challenging when you are working with more than one student, as the students' desire to stay with one activity may vary. Again, this is an opportunity to encourage communication to indicate being "all done," or to teach a student to "wait a minute." Whenever possible, you should comply with an individual's requests by allowing the student to leave the group (perhaps after completing one more task, if increasing time in the group is a goal) or by providing the student with an alternative activity or choice within the activity. For example, imagine that the group is learning to identify words, and each student is choosing a favorite picture to match with sight words. Piper no longer wants to match pictures to words. First, provide her with a choice of different pictures (perhaps including some simpler words to help her feel more successful). If this does not interest Piper, ask her to collect the pictures from the group, providing her with an alternative activity for a short break. Try making the possible reinforcement more clear by allowing her to "drive" her completed word–picture match on a train. Finally, if you are unable to maintain her interest in this activity, present a choice of two alternative activities (e.g., a word identification program on the computer, or word identification while reading a book with a paraprofessional). Again, it may take time for students to learn to stick with activities.

Incorporate Turn Taking

Turn taking between/among students can be used to increase modeling of appropriate behavior, to maintain attention, and to provide students with opportunities to choose what they would like to do when their turn comes around. For example, when learning to complete a puzzle, students may each take a turn placing their preferred piece into the larger puzzle. Students may even be able to help each other figure out where specific pieces go. Or one student may have the pieces, and other students may need to ask for the pieces they want. During a cooking activity, students may take turns measuring and pouring. You can continue to take turns as well, modeling appropriate or more advanced behavior and language during group activities.

Group Instruction

Incorporate Your Students' Preferred Materials

When the entire group needs to engage in the same activity, allowing individual students choice becomes challenging, if not impossible. For many lessons, it may be possible to have the group choose the activity or pieces of an activity. For example, the group can choose stories or songs for circle time. This may be done cooperatively, or students may rotate who gets to choose. You may find specific activities or topics that a majority of the class enjoys, such as cooking, a recent movie, or rocket ships, and those themes can then be used in whole-group activities for teaching a variety of lessons. If you are unable to incorporate student choice into the activity, you may need to consider whether or not CPRT is an appropriate strategy for that activity.

Follow Your Students' Lead

Some of the strategies listed above can be used when a single student wishes to change activities. However, if the group appears to be losing interest in the activity and many students are not paying attention, it may be time to "switch things around." This can be done through changing the way the activity is being conducted, increasing animation, allowing students to choose some aspect of the activity, or putting the lesson away and beginning something new. Anticipating the need for a change is important, so that the group does not receive a reward for inappropriate behavior. Be sure that the group as a whole is asking appropriately for a change. This can be done simply by observing the students; however, you may have a (previously taught) signal that students can use to request a change, such as raising a card. If a student requests a change, the group can be polled by asking all the students who want a change to use the signal. This allows students to attend to the lesson while still being able to ask for a change.

Incorporate Turn Taking

You can model appropriate behavior for the group by joining in group activities.

Taking a turn at the activity in which your students are engaged—whether this is creating an art project, eating a snack, or completing a math worksheet—gives students an important model for appropriate behavior. Additionally, larger-group activities may provide opportunities for cooperative action rather than traditional turn taking. For example, the entire group may need to follow instructions for using a parachute. The group can work together to bounce balls on the parachute or make a tunnel. Students can choose whether they wish to shake the parachute or go under the tunnel, and then take turns doing the other action. Similarly, small subgroups facilitated by a student leader or paraprofessional can also take turns. For example, each group can represent an animal, and the leader can have the groups take turns by doing their animal sounds and actions or by watching their classmates do the same. Teams can take turns completing math problems or acting out a story.

COMPONENT 5: MULTIPLE CUES (BROADENING ATTENTION)

Use multiple examples of materials and concepts to ensure broad understanding.

Group activities offer a perfect opportunity to teach using multiple examples of materials and concepts, as you may not have iden-

tical sets of objects for every student. Using multiple cues (i.e., conditional discriminations) for students who are specifically overselective can also be adapted for use during group instruction, although it may take some planning.

Targeting Individuals within a Group

Use Multiple Examples

Various examples of certain materials and concepts can easily be incorporated into group activities. Some of this variation may already naturally occur in the materials you have available in your classroom. For example, if a student is required to ask for scissors during an art activity, you are likely to have several pairs of scissors that do not all look identical. By giving the student a different pair of scissors each time, you are broadening his attention to the concept of *scissors* as something you cut with (the feature that all scissors share), rather than *scissors* as one specific pair or as some irrelevant aspect (e.g., the color or size of the handles). Additionally, multiple concepts can be taught using the same materials, so that the student learns to respond to the appropriate element. If students in a small group are playing with blocks, you may ask a student to count the blocks, and then later ask her to sort them into color groups. Thus you are teaching counting, color identification, and sorting with the same set of materials, ensuring that the student can respond to each of these various elements.

Incorporate Conditional Discriminations

You can use multiple cues with individuals within a small group in the same manner as you would with students on an individual basis. Often in small groups you may have some students who are ready to learn multiple cues, as well as students who are not ready (i.e., students whose developmental age is under 36 months). With students who are ready, you can present a task related to the overall group activity that also requires response to multiple cues. For example, if you are working with a small group during an art activity, a student can be asked to give a peer a large piece of red paper when there are both large and small pieces of paper that are red, blue, and green. When your group is identifying the weather during circle time, one student can simply choose a raindrop when it is rainy. A more advanced student may need to discriminate between the kind of weather you are having and the amount. For example, one raindrop versus a cluster of several raindrops indicates a little rain or a lot of rain, and one cloud versus a cluster of several clouds indicates one cloud or a lot of clouds in the sky. You can also present instructions and require a response on the basis of multiple cues. While reading a story to your class about a boy dressing himself, ask Naakai to point to a peer who is wearing a blue shirt. Since there will be shirts, pants, socks, and shoes of different colors, Naakai's choice must be based on both color and article of clothing.

Group Instruction

Use Multiple Examples

Providing each student in a group with slightly different materials for the same activity or concept is an excellent way to incorporate multiple examples into group activities. For example, a group of students learning to identify states from a map of the United States may all be given a slightly different map. Providing students with different materials also creates a practical opportunity to work on social skills, as they share with each other how their materials are different. Another option to broaden

attention may be to pose different questions to students about multiple features of the materials. For example, you may ask one student what color paper she would like, and another student whether he would like a large or a small piece of paper.

Incorporate Conditional Discriminations

With a group as a whole, working on multiple cues is most appropriate when the majority of students are developmentally ready for this type of teaching. Games and activities can be altered to provide instructions with multiple components. For example, a game of "musical shapes" can be used, in which students need to stand on the blue squares (not the blue circles or red squares) when the music stops. When students are asked to write their names on their papers, they may need to choose the green pencil from the many choices of crayons and pencils on their desks.

**COMPONENT 6:
DIRECT REINFORCEMENT**

Provide reinforcement that is naturally or directly related to the activity or behavior.

Targeting Individuals within a Group

Throughout the school day, you have multiple opportunities to require student behavior that can be reinforced in a direct or natural way. For example, a student may want to get some scissors from the cupboard, go to the rest room, or play with a toy on a high shelf. These are all opportunities to provide direct reinforcement for appropriate language use. Finding direct reinforcers can be more complicated for academic tasks. Incorporating favorite items in the tasks can be helpful.

For example, learning to count trains can lead to playing with trains. Copying letters related to a favorite movie title may be rewarded with being allowed to talk about the movie with a classmate. Placing the date on the calendar after naming the number may be rewarding for some students.

Group Instruction

Similar to the difficulties in following the group's lead and providing choices, finding direct reinforcers that are motivating for the entire group may take some thinking. For example, if your students like movement, and you want to work on counting, the whole class can count the number of times one student jumps. All students who participate in the counting can then jump that many times as a reward. If the class members have chosen a story about a character or theme they enjoy, they can be rewarded for good listening when you turn the page and go on with the story.

Consider what your students enjoy and how you can use those activities to reward skills you want them to learn.

**COMPONENT 7:
CONTINGENT CONSEQUENCE
(IMMEDIATE AND APPROPRIATE)**

Present consequences immediately, based on the students' responses.

Your responses should be contingent upon student behavior, whether you are working individually with a student or when working with a group. The potential reward should be clear to the student or group of students before the activity begins.

Targeting Individuals within a Group

When a student in a group behaves appropriately by responding correctly or making a reasonable attempt, you should provide a reward. When a student in a group is behaving incorrectly or inappropriately, you can ask the student to try again or can withhold a reward. If another student in the group (who is not working directly with you) does something appropriate (e.g., spontaneously asks for a new crayon), that student can also be rewarded for the appropriate behavior. Likewise, inappropriate behavior should not be rewarded, even with attention.

If you cannot provide an immediate reward because you are working with another student, acknowledge the request and come back to it when you can.

Group Instruction

When the entire group is behaving appropriately, reinforcement should be provided immediately and clearly to the group, just as it would be with individual students. For example, if everyone participates in the class spelling bee, they can watch excerpts from a movie about a spelling bee. If the entire group is not responding correctly or is behaving inappropriately, then a reward should not be delivered, and the group should be asked to try again. If specific students are trying hard or responding appropriately while other students are not listening, reward those students who are doing a good job. Then give the group as a whole a chance to try again or to earn a new reward. The students receiving reinforcement for appropriate behavior provide a nice model for the other students. If a student is having particular difficulty, additional prompts or supports may be needed to increase success in the group environment.

COMPONENT 8: REINFORCEMENT OF ATTEMPTS

Reward good trying to encourage your students to try again in the future.

Targeting Individuals within a Group

If you are expecting a specific response from each student in the group, reward reasonable, goal-directed attempts at correct responding. For example, if a student is learning to write letters and attempts to draw the letter *A* but is quite messy, you might still reward him for trying and then assist him with making his next attempt closer to the correct response. Of course, the type of response that is considered good trying for this student (a messy letter *A*) may not be considered good trying for another student, who has been writing the letter *A* well for months and is now working on writing words. It is okay to reward different behavior for different students in the same group when they have varying skill levels.

Remember that an attempt is a behavior that serves the same function as the target skill, without the accuracy or clarity of a "correct" response.

Group Instruction

When the entire group is responding appropriately, some students may be responding perfectly (e.g., imitating hand movements in a song), while others are observing and trying but not doing quite as well (e.g., following half of the motions). If the students are trying hard, they can be rewarded with the rest of the group (e.g., standing in front with you to lead the song). If the group is working on a cooperative activity, such as making a banner for a class presentation, and the students are working hard but need some assistance to make the writing clear, reward the small steps and "good trying" as they work together to move the project forward.

Chapter Summary

The components of CPRT can be adapted for use during group activities. The same basic principles of ABA are still in effect. Some additional planning may be needed to adapt activities to include some of the components of CPRT when you are working with multiple students. Continue to use motivating strategies, such as allowing students to choose the activity as a group, or modifying the activity to allow some choice within the activity. Attention may be difficult for some students in a group setting, so modify the expectations by allowing students to build tolerance for group activities or by asking another adult to assist with providing clear instructions to specific students. Provide instructions at different levels, depending on the needs of various students in the group. Vary your expectations based on the students' skill levels, and allow students at different levels to be models for each other. Incorporate turn taking between/among students whenever possible. Notice which activities a majority of the class find fun and engaging, and use those materials or activities to teach various lessons. Reward the entire group for working together toward a common goal, even if not all students have mastered the task. One of the benefits of CPRT is that it structures group activities in a way that increases motivation for all students in the group, which will help improve attention and participation in the activity.

CHAPTER 5
Meeting Individual Goals Using CPRT

CHAPTER OVERVIEW

CPRT can be used to address Individualized Education Program (IEP) goals as well as standards in curriculum areas. You can incorporate CPRT to teach toward existing goals, as well as to create new goals with CPRT in mind. It may be helpful to use CPRT with groups of students with similar goals. CPRT can be used to teach communication, object play, social interaction, and academic skills.

The following sections are included:

Addressing IEP and Curriculum Goals Using CPRT
    Writing IEP Goals
    Implementing IEP Goals and Addressing Curriculum Areas

Communication Skills
    Where to Begin
    When to Teach
    How to Move Forward

Object Play Skills
    Where to Begin
    When to Teach
    How to Move Forward

Social Interaction Skills
    Where to Begin
    When to Teach
    How to Move Forward

Academic Skills
    Where to Begin
    When to Teach
    How to Move Forward

This chapter has a corresponding training lecture on the DVD accompanying this manual (*CPRT Session 3: CPRT with Groups and for Student Goals*).

Now that you understand the steps of CPRT and know how to use those steps both with an individual student and with a group, it is time to think about teaching specific skills with CPRT. CPRT can be used to teach a variety of skills. This chapter emphasizes the practical aspects of using CPRT to teach various skills.

 For more information about the research showing the effectiveness of these strategies for teaching each curriculum area, see *Chapter 9*.

Addressing IEP and Curriculum Goals Using CPRT

An **Individualized Education Program (IEP)** is created to meet the unique educational needs of a specific student and is required in the United States by the Individuals with Disabilities Education Improvement Act of 2004. Although there are some general rules about how to write IEP goals, programs often differ in the way they write goals. You may find that students join your class with a wide variety of learning goals, and that these are written to be implemented and measured in different ways. These factors make your job complicated!

In addition to meeting IEP goals, students need to learn the standards-based curriculum in your classroom. We have provided examples of how to use CPRT to address areas such as communication, object play skills, social interaction skills, and academics for your students with autism.

Writing IEP Goals

As you become more comfortable with using CPRT to educate your students, you will want to be mindful of these strategies when developing IEP goals for further learning.

- *Write goals to address generalization of skills.* The eventual goal is for students to learn to use their skills in a variety of settings, with many people. CPRT is designed to be used in natural learning environments and to draw upon natural cues in a student's environment. For example, if the student's needs require a goal that targets an appropriate response to yes–no questions, consider the times of day when this will be both a functional skill for the student and one that has a natural reinforcer. Think about different people with whom the skill might be functional. Answering yes–no questions in response to needs or wants (e.g., "Do you need to go to the bathroom?" or "Do you want a turn?") is a more naturalistic use of this skill than answering yes–no questions in response to factual queries that may not be of interest to the student or may not have a natural reinforcer (e.g., "Is this a zebra?" or "Is Kevin wearing a blue shirt?"). This will promote generalization, so the student can use this new skill at home and in the community.

- *Write goals to target spontaneous, independent skill use.* One of the goals of CPRT for all students is their spontaneous and independent use of the skills they learn. Initially, it may be helpful and necessary to provide support as a student learns a new skill. However, it is important to write goals that include spontaneous, independent demonstration of the skill. This is the best indication that your student will be able to use the skill independently and functionally outside your classroom. For example, you may want to increase the complexity of your student's requests and comments by having the student use an adjective and noun together (e.g., "a big dog," "the princess sticker"). Write the goal to focus on the student's independent response to what he sees in his environment. Instead of the student's responding to questions such as "What do you want?" or "What do you see?" as the final goal, target the student's learning to spontaneously request objects or describe things in the environment.

- *Write goals reflecting teaching activities that work well in your classroom.* You probably already have ideas about when CPRT will be best incorporated into your daily classroom activities. Keep this in mind as you develop specific goals for your students. If a student needs to learn to interact with peers, and you facilitate play between your students and their typically developing peers during snack time and outside play, write the goal so that it can be targeted during these activities. For example, you can teach your student to ask independently for more juice from a peer during snack time, and to respond when a peer asks for more raisins. If you do a cooking activity with your students on a weekly basis, you might teach subtraction of fractions in a naturalistic way. If you intend to pose the question "The recipe requires ½ cup of flour, and I just added ¼ cup of flour. How much more do I need?", the goal might be written as follows: "Michael will demonstrate addition and subtraction of basic fractions with 80% accuracy throughout the school day."

Implementing IEP Goals and Addressing Curriculum Areas

Goals for multiple students of varying skill levels can be addressed together by using CPRT. CPRT can and should be used throughout the school day, in art, circle time, meal time, literacy, math, and other teacher-directed activities. *Tables 5.1, 5.2, and 5.3* describe three sets of student profiles and accompanying goals. Consider the students with these profiles and goals as a sample of the students who might be in

your classroom. The outlines accompanying these tables indicate how all the students' goals are incorporated into group activities. (First review the tables, then go to the outlines.) For each example, assume that the student has an educational classification of autism, and that reinforcing activities and items have been determined ahead of time. Each set of profiles and examples targets a different age group: preschool (*Table 5.1*), kindergarten–first grade (*Table 5.2*), and second–third grades (*Table 5.3*).

Preschool: Michelle, Bryan, and Kalea (Table 5.1)

USING CPRT AT CIRCLE TIME

Activity: Circle time

Materials: Animal puppets, printed student names, pocket chart with student photographs, color book, and corresponding objects

"Hello Song": The teacher begins by singing the "Hello Song," which incorporates several animal sounds. She takes a turn and sings the first part of each sentence; she then pauses to allow the students to fill in the sound of the animal at the end (acquisition skill for Michelle and Bryan; maintenance skill for Kalea). When they are successful, she allows them to pet her puppet of the animal that makes that sound (direct reinforcer).

> **Kalea:** The teacher then asks Kalea to sing the last line independently (acquisition skill; Goal 1). Kalea sings, " ... and I say hello!" The teacher exclaims, "You sang that just right!" and allows Kalea to choose the next song.

Attendance Chart: The teacher holds up the pocket chart with photographs of the students and their name cards. She says, "I have some pictures."

TABLE 5.1. Scenario 1: Preschool

This table presents student profiles and accompanying goals for three students in a preschool classroom.

Student profile	IEP goals or curriculum areas
Michelle is a 3-year-old girl attending a special day preschool class. She currently has no intelligible speech, but she can exchange single pictures for highly desired items and tries to imitate single words. She points to items to request them, and uses sounds and some word approximations when a picture is not available. Michelle enjoys music and especially loves a classroom number song that is used at circle time, her favorite activity during the day. She likes to look at clocks and numbers, and is just beginning to try to count. She demonstrates understanding of rote counting to 5 by touching each number as it is being named. She is able to wait to take turns with her peers, remains seated for up to 15 minutes, and enjoys choosing some of the activities used at circle time. Michelle is learning her colors and shapes.	1. Michelle will indicate that she wants a turn at an activity by using a verbalization, gesture, or picture exchange during 80% of requests on 4 of 5 days. 2. Michelle will use single-word approximations to ask for objects, food, or play opportunities, 5 times within each school day on 4 consecutive measurement days. 3. Michelle will be able to count independently to 5 using word approximations when she is presented with an opportunity to count (either in the classroom or on the playground) on 4 of 5 opportunities. 4. Michelle will independently sort, match, or point to named colors and shapes on 8 out of 10 opportunities.
Bryan is an almost 4-year-old boy with emerging language skills. He uses many single words to express his wants and needs, but has difficulty putting two words together. He often needs a visual prompt to use language. He attends a special day class with six peers. Bryan loves cars and trucks; if left to himself, he would play with them all day. He likes to do puzzles, paint, and use Play-Doh. He repeats the names of colors and shapes, which he knows receptively. He can count by rote to 10, but does not yet show understanding of quantity. Bryan prefers to play alone and will often lash out at another student who tries to join him in play.	1. Bryan will use one or two words to spontaneously request objects, toys, or activities a minimum of 10 times throughout the school day on 4 of 5 days. 2. Bryan will independently name 10 colors and 5 shapes with 100% accuracy, when requested by an adult, on 4 of 5 days. 3. Bryan will demonstrate understanding of quantity by matching objects to numerals up to 5 when given the appropriate materials on 8 of 10 opportunities. 4. Bryan will allow a peer to play near him without protesting, and will share materials/toys with that peer (with adults facilitating and creating opportunities for engagement), for up to 10 minutes over 3 days.
Kalea is a 5-year-old attending preschool 4 days a week in a special day class. She has many preacademic skills and a large single-word vocabulary; she can also independently use one or two words to request. Kalea tries to sing along with songs during music and circle times, but usually is just using any words she currently knows and not the appropriate lyrics. She adores flowers and will request them throughout the day. She will often give one of her artificial flowers to another student. She is starting to pretend by "sniffing" or watering a flower, but is not yet putting steps together or using other toys in pretend play. She can count to 20 and understands the concept of matching quantity to number. She likes to paint and color. Kalea does not use adjectives to describe what she wants or sees. She will take turns with adult facilitation, but does not know how to get others to join in play with her.	1. Kalea will be able to sing the appropriate lyrics to 2–4 familiar classroom songs during circle time, with 80% accuracy, on 4 of 5 school days. 2. Kalea will independently use 2- or 3-word phrases to request objects or describe what she sees, using adjective(s) + noun (e.g., "the blue car"), with 80% accuracy on 4 of 5 opportunities. 3. Kalea will initiate interaction with other children when presented with appropriate stimuli or social situations, and will maintain an interaction for 2 exchanges, in 3 of 4 opportunities at least once per day. 4. Kalea will spontaneously engage in 2-step symbolic play actions with preferred materials during 80% of opportunities over 4 of 5 days.

Bryan: Bryan raises his hand. The teacher says, "What do you want, Bryan?" He replies, "Turn" (Goal 1). She rewards this maintenance skill by allowing him to pick out his name and place it next to his picture in the chart.

Michelle: After Bryan sits back down, the teacher looks at Michelle and asks, "Do you want a turn?" Michelle does not respond. The teacher gains Michelle's attention and asks again. Michelle responds by patting her chest to indicate that she would like a turn. The teacher models saying, "Turn." Michelle says, "urn" (acquisition skill; Goals 1 and 2). To reward this attempt, the teacher gives Michelle her name card to place.

Story: Next, the teacher takes out a book about colors and corresponding objects, and lays out colored objects on the floor. She names the colors as she does so—a red squishy ball, a blue light toy, a purple stuffed Barney doll, and a green plastic lizard. As she turns each page in the book, she sings, "The [object] is [color name] …"

Michelle: The teacher asks Michelle to pick the toy that is the same color as the red page (Goal 4). The teacher shows her two different objects, and she chooses the red ball and places it on the page. "Yes, that's red," says the teacher, and she gives Michelle the red squishy ball.

Bryan: Next, she asks who wants a turn. Bryan says, "Turn." She models the phrase "My turn" for him to repeat. When he does, she allows him to match the colors. Then, pointing to the next page (blue), she asks Bryan, "What color is this?" He replies, "Blue" (Goal 2), and she gives him the blue light toy. Now the teacher takes a turn, matching a new color that the students haven't learned. "Look," she says. "I'm matching the brown bear sticker to the brown page."

Kalea: While the teacher is taking a turn, Kalea tries to grab the book. The teacher redirects Kalea; when she is sitting nicely, the teacher asks her, "What color do you want?" Kalea responds with "Purple." The teacher rewards the attempt by giving her the purple Barney doll. Then the teacher shows a new page and says, "Say the whole sentence. What color do you want?" Kalea says, "Give me the green one" (Goal 2). The teacher praises her effort and gives her the green lizard. After Kalea has a moment to play, the teacher collects all the colored items and assesses the students' motivation by asking, "Who wants more of the color game?"

USING CPRT AT ART TIME

Activity: Art time

Materials: Colored shape stickers, corresponding shapes drawn on white paper

Transition from Circle: It is time to leave circle and sit down at the art table.

Kalea: The teacher tells Kalea, "It is time for art. Tell your friends to come with you to art." Kalea looks at Michelle and says nothing. The teacher models saying, "Michelle and Bryan, come to art!" Kalea says, "Come to art" (Goal 3). The teacher lets Kalea lead the way to the art table and choose her seat.

At the Art Table: The teacher seats Bryan next to Kalea, so that Kalea can pass materials to Bryan and he can share the supplies with her (Goal 4). The teacher explains that today's activity is matching shapes. All the students must ask for the colored sticker they need to complete their paper. Because all the students enjoy stickers, this activity has a built-in natural reinforcer. The teacher shows them the paper and names each colored shape. Then she shows them the stickers and again names the colors and shapes for them. She uses her own paper to take turns modeling language and the activity.

Bryan: After passing out the paper, the teacher turns to Bryan and asks him which colored shape he would like first. He responds with "Green." She replies, "Green what?" He says, "I want green circle." (Goals 1 and 2). She gives him the requested sticker.

Kalea: The teacher tells Kalea to ask Bryan what colored shape he is gluing on his paper. Kalea looks at Bryan and says his name. The teacher says, "Bryan, what shape is that?" Kalea imitates the teacher and asks him the shape (Goal 3). He tells her it is a square. The teacher prompts Kalea to say, "Hooray, Bryan!" Kalea then gets to choose the shape she wants to put on her paper.

Michelle: The teacher asks Michelle to point to the correct colored shape from a choice of three (Goal 4). Michelle points, and then takes the sticker and puts it on her paper.

Kalea: The teacher asks Kalea to tell Michelle the name of the color/shape on her paper (Goal 2). Kalea correctly labels the blue triangle and then gets a blue triangle for her own paper as well. Lastly, the teacher helps Michelle hold up two stickers, and Kalea points to one. The teacher tells her to ask. Kalea responds by saying, "I will stick the yellow circle" (Goal 2).

The activity continues, with the students taking turns and choosing colored shapes from one another with the teacher's help, for as long as the stickers remain motivating. Bryan loses interest in the shapes first, so the teacher offers animal stickers, which he enjoys. Instead of asking him to label the shape he will get from the teacher, she asks him to label the shape on which he puts the animal sticker.

Note: You could also easily target multiple cue discriminations during this activity if it is an appropriate skill for the students in your group.

USING CPRT AT SNACK TIME

Activity: Snack time

Materials: Cups, napkins, apple juice, clear containers of multicolored goldfish crackers, raisins, apple slices, and pretzels

At the Snack Table: The students are sitting at the snack table, and the teacher is sitting opposite them. A cup and an open napkin are in front of each student. The teacher takes a turn first and models saying, "Yum, I want to eat apples."

Kalea: The teacher looks at Kalea and waits. Kalea tells her, "Eat goldfish." Since this is spontaneous, the teacher gives Kalea one goldfish. Kalea reaches for more, and the teacher asks her, "What do you want?" Kalea replies, "Green" (maintenance skill), to which the teacher replies, "You want a green what?" (acquisition skill). Kalea tells her, "A green fish, please!"(Goal 2). The teacher smiles at her and says, "Here is your green goldfish."

Bryan: The teacher turns to Bryan and asks him what he would like. He says, "Raisins." "How many?" the teacher asks. Bryan says, "Lots!" The teacher lays out raisins one at a time in front of Bryan and asks him to count each one as she places it on the table. He counts, "1, 2, 3, 4, 5" (Goal 3). She gives him the raisins, saying, "Five is a lot!"

Michelle: Michelle reaches for the container with the pretzels in it. The teacher models the word for her, and Michelle says, "Pretz" (Goal 2). The teacher gives her one pretzel to reinforce her good attempt, and then says, "Okay, count them while I give them to you." She lays three more pretzels in front of Michelle and has her point to each one as she counts them out loud (Goal 3).

Kindergarten–First Grade: José, Sara, and Darren (Table 5.2)

USING CPRT AT LANGUAGE ARTS

Activity: Letter and word recognition

Materials: Letter cards, character stickers, writing/matching boards for students, toy animals

The students, José, Sara, and Darren, are seated at a small round table with the teacher. She reviews the alphabet with the students by showing them letter cards of all the letters and naming them.

> **José:** The teacher shows José a letter card. "What letter is this, José?" She holds up an *S*. José looks at it and says, "*S*" (Goal 1). "Good," says the teacher; she gives him the letter, which has a Superman sticker on it (he likes superheroes).

Next, the teacher takes a turn and models a more advanced skill. She writes *all* on her whiteboard and places the *B* card in front of it. "*B* goes with *a-l-l* to spell *ball*."

> **Sara:** Sara is working on *at* words (e.g., *bat, cat, hat*) and has a board with a blank space followed by *at*. The teacher asks Sara if *B* can be put in front of *at* to make a word. Sara looks at her board and puts the *B* in front. "What does it say, Sara?" Sara replies, "*B-at. Bat!*" (acquisition skill, Goal 1). "That's great," the teacher tells her, "it spells *bat!*" She asks Sara whether she would like to take another turn or share her letter with Darren. Sara chooses to give the letter to Darren (Goal 3).

> **Darren:** Darren has a matching board for the capital letters. He places the *B* from Sara on the correct corresponding letter (Goal 1). He is rewarded by being allowed to choose a toy animal whose name begins with the same letter to play with.

The teacher continues the lesson in this manner, allowing José to name the letters (he is rewarded with the embedded stickers), Sara to test them with the *at* board (she is rewarded by allowing her to choose to take a turn or share), and Darren to match them to his board (he is rewarded with animal toys whose names begin with the same letter he is matching). The teacher models as needed and gives praise throughout the session.

USING CPRT AT MATH

Activity: Number recognition, addition–subtraction

Materials: Number cards, addition–subtraction folder templates (three squares printed horizontally with + or – and an = between them)

The teacher shows and labels each number card, and allows the students the choice of whispering or yelling as they repeat each number after her (maintenance skill). She knows that "being the teacher" is motivating for all her students, so she uses this role to reinforce the students' behavior during a math activity.

> **Darren:** The teacher holds up two numbers (3 and 5) and says, "Darren, tell us what numbers these are" (Goal 3). He labels both numbers correctly, and she gives him the corresponding number cards and says, "Okay, Darren is the teacher."

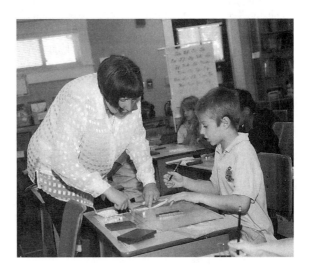

TABLE 5.2. Scenario 2: Kindergarten–First Grade

This table presents student profiles and accompanying goals for three students in a kindergarten and first-grade classroom.

Student profile	IEP goals or curriculum areas
José is a 6-year-old boy who attends a K–1 special day class. He has some intelligible phrase speech, which he uses to request and at times to comment, but he does not yet use sentences. He can match uppercase letters but does not name them. José is at the beginning level of reading sight words. José counts to 20 and can give objects up to 10 from a field of 12–15 with 80% accuracy. He requires visuals to augment learning. José has difficulty interacting with other students and is often alone on the playground and at lunch.	1. José will name the uppercase letters when they are presented in random order, with 100% accuracy, on 4 of 5 opportunities. 2. José will demonstrate the ability to complete addition sums in single digits, with visual support, during 4 of 5 opportunities. 3. Within 1 school year, José will spontaneously use simple sentences 5 times in each school day on 6 out of 8 days. 4. José will join a group appropriately (by spontaneously waving, saying hello, asking to play, etc.), and will remain in proximity to other students during small-group activities and lunch, for 15 minutes over 4 of 5 school days.
Sara is a first grader in the same special day class as José. She is a 7-year-old girl who uses five- to six-word sentences but does not always express herself well to get her needs met. Sara knows all of the upper- and lower-case alphabet, as well as the sound each letter makes. She is learning to recognize simple words in print. She prints her first and last names. Sara knows how to do addition for single-digit numbers. She is currently working on subtraction skills. Although Sara has many friends, she still has difficulty sharing materials during class activities.	1. Sara will decode simple consonant–vowel–consonant words when shown a variety of printed materials, with 8 out of 10 words correct as measured by interim assessment on 4 out of 5 occasions. 2. Sara will demonstrate the ability to do single-digit subtraction problems independently, with at least 80% correct, on 4 of 5 school days. 3. When Sara is at an activity with plenty of materials, she will be able to share with her peers spontaneously for up to 5 turns on 4 of 5 school days.
Darren is a first grader. He primarily uses gestures to communicate and makes some inconsistent attempts at single words. He is able to use a picture exchange communication system to make requests with an open-handed prompt. Darren sings the ABC song by rote (using approximations), but does not recognize the letters of the alphabet. Darren counts by rote to 5 (using approximations), but has not yet developed numeral recognition. Darren engages in parallel play near peers, but he has little to no interaction with them. He is often alone and ignores those around him.	1. Darren will match the letters of the uppercase alphabet when given 2 sets of letters, with 100% accuracy, on 4 of 5 opportunities. 2. Darren will point to the requested numerals up to 10, with 100% accuracy, during 4 of 5 opportunities. 3. Darren will use words or pictures to communicate at least 20 times without prompting throughout the school day to request objects/activities on 4 of 5 school days. 4. Darren will interact with peers during structured play by taking turns and sharing materials during daily activities, with teacher facilitation, on 70% of opportunities on 3 days.

She helps Darren pass out the numbers. He chooses to give the number 3 to José and the number 5 to Sara (Goal 4). Next, the teacher holds up two more numbers (1 and 2) for Darren and asks, "Where is number 2?" Darren takes the 2 card and, smiling, gives it to Sara (Goals 2 and 4). The teacher wants to reward his spontaneous sharing. "That was great, Darren!" she says. "You picked the correct number and even gave it to Sara without being asked! You may choose two animals."

Sara: Sara's folder has a subtraction sign between the first two boxes. The teacher tells Sara, "Put your number 5 here" (pointing to the first box), "and your number 2 here" (pointing to the second box). She then asks, "What is the answer?" and points to the third box. Sara says, "Five minus two equals three." The teacher announces, "Great job! Now Sara is the teacher." With the teacher's help, Sara gives José the number 2 card and tells him to do his math problem.

José: José makes a nice attempt by reading the numbers on his folder without solving the problem (Goal 2). The teacher praises his effort, and he is allowed to flick the number cards with his fingers. The teacher says, "Now I will take a turn," and solves an addition problem on another folder.

The lesson continues in this manner until math time is over.

Second–Third Grades: Max, Patrick, and Joy (Table 5.3)

USING CPRT IN A SOCIAL SKILLS ACTIVITY

Activity: Playing a game with peers

Materials: Several fun, interesting tactile balls in a bucket; chairs in a circle (several more chairs than students), with pictures of animals pasted on colored paper on the backs of the chairs.

Animal Game: As students come to the circle, each student chooses a chair/animal. The teacher announces, "We are going to play a new ball game today!"

Joy: The teacher shows Joy the bucket of balls and asks, "Joy, which ball should we use?" (Goal 2). Joy says, "The green squishy ball!" The teacher lets Joy pick the ball out of the container and hand it to her.

The teacher throws the ball in the air several times to gain students' attention. She holds up a small whiteboard that has the rules of the game written on it, and she reads each step aloud:

1. Catch the ball.
2. Look at a friend.
3. Tell your friend to find a color and an animal.
4. Wait until your friend finds the right chair.
5. Wait until your friend looks at you and says, "Give me the ball!"
6. Give the ball to your friend any way you choose (throw it high or low, roll the ball, bounce the ball).

Patrick: The teacher starts the game by saying, "Patrick, go to the red elephant chair!" Patrick responds by sitting in a chair with a red lion on it. The teacher states, "You found a red lion chair. Where is the red elephant?" while pointing to the correct chair. Once Patrick moves to the correct chair, the teacher waits expectantly until he looks at her and mumbles, "Give ... ball." She reinforces his attempt at communication by throwing the ball to him. Patrick then says, "Max, yellow chair," but he is difficult to understand and is speaking quickly. The teacher speaks slowly and says, "Try again." Patrick slowly says, "Max, go to the yellow frog chair" (Goal 1).

Max: Max does not respond to Patrick, and so the teacher walks over to him and points to Patrick. Patrick repeats his sentence, and the teacher takes a step toward the appropriate chair. Max follows and then finds the correct chair (Goal 4). Patrick waits for Max to ask for the ball (Goal 2). Patrick bounces it to him (direct reinforcement for his turn). The teacher looks at Max and says, "What happened!?"; Max replies, "He threw the ball" (Goal 1). Max then takes his turn at the game (direct reinforcement).

TABLE 5.3. Scenario 3: Second–Third Grades

This table presents student profiles and accompanying goals for three students in a second- and third-grade classroom.

Student profile	IEP goals or curriculum areas
Max is a 7-year-old boy who attends a grade 2–3 special education class. He makes requests using full sentences, but he has trouble maintaining eye contact and rarely answers questions or makes comments. Max loves to read and is reading well above grade level, though it is difficult for him to talk about things he has read or recall details. During free time and recess, Max typically reads his book and ignores invitations from other students to talk or play games.	1. Max will use sentences to comment or answer questions 5–10 times in each school day, on at least 8 out of 10 occasions, with both staff and peers. 2. Max will use eye contact in coordination with language as is appropriate to the situation on 4 of 5 opportunities. 3. When given a short story at his grade level, Max will verbally identify 2 main ideas in the story on 4 out of 5 opportunities. 4. Max will respond to initiations from his same-age peers by participating in a conversation or collaborative activity for at least 10 minutes on 4 of 5 school days.
Patrick is a third grader in the same class as Max. He can adequately express his needs and make comments, but he often mumbles or speaks too quickly to be understood, in order to escape the social situation. Patrick is reading at grade level and is learning to identify different types of sentences. Patrick has difficulty working independently on tasks and often needs constant supervision to complete an assignment. Although he appears interested in observing his peers, he often leaves activities that require direct interaction with peers.	1. Patrick will use appropriate articulation and rate of speech in sentence production on 4 of 5 opportunities across 5 school days. 2. Patrick will accurately identify declarative, exclamatory, imperative, and interrogative sentences in a grade-level text, with 8 out of 10 correct for each type, on 3 school days. 3. Patrick will begin work within 1 minute of teacher instruction and continue working for 10 minutes, with only visual prompts, on 3 school days. 4. Patrick will remain with a group of students and participate in an interactive activity for 10 minutes on 4 of 5 school days.
Joy is an 8-year-old girl who enjoys animals. She prefers to speak exclusively about animals and has difficulty using expanded sentences related to other topics. She will often inappropriately introduce the topic of animals rather than respond to non-animal-related initiations from others, particularly when called on by the teacher to answer a question. She enjoys telling stories, but they often do not make sense or follow a logical sequence. Joy will interact with her peers if she is able to direct the activity, but she has trouble participating in structured games with specified rules where she is required to follow directions from another. She is reading below grade level and has difficulty keeping track of details in stories.	1. Joy will engage in appropriate conversations by selecting, maintaining, and closing conversation topics chosen by a teacher or another student during 80% of opportunities. 2. Joy will answer or attempt to answer open-ended questions on a variety of topics (unrelated to animals) on 4 of 5 opportunities across 5 school days. 3. Joy will identify the beginning, middle, and end of a story on 3 school days. 4. Joy will follow rules in structured games, as measured by cooperative participation, for at least 15 minutes on 4 of 5 school days.

Patrick: After several more turns, the teacher asks Patrick if he would like to take a break after his next turn, because he has stayed with the group so nicely (Goal 4). Patrick gets the ball and says, "Ms. Smith, go to the red lion chair!" The teacher walks to the chair and says, "Patrick, throw me the ball!" She catches the ball, and Patrick is allowed to sit on a chair away from the group.

Joy: The teacher then says, "Joy, go to the orange walrus chair," and Joy replies, "No, I want to go to the yellow frog chair." The teacher prompts Joy to go to the appropriate chair (Goal 4) and complete her turn, and then tells Joy, "You can choose a new ball to throw and the chair you want to throw it from!" as a reward for completing the structured aspect of the activity. Joy chooses a new ball and chair and says, "There's a frog on that chair. Frogs are amphibious and … " The teacher says, "You want to talk about frogs, but we are all waiting for the ball." Joy replies, "We're throwing a blue light-up ball" (Goal 1), and then selects a peer and finishes her turn.

The game continues in this manner, with everyone taking turns (including the teacher). Students are rewarded as part of the game by choosing materials and method of tossing the ball, getting to ask questions, and so on, depending on what motivates each of them.

USING CPRT IN A READING ACTIVITY

Activity: Reading a short story

Materials: Several books and manipulative toys associated with each story

The students are sitting at the small reading table, with the teacher facing them.

Joy: The teacher turns to Joy and asks, "What book should we read today?" and holds up several choices (Goal 2, maintenance skill). Joy selects *Frog and Toad Are Friends*, and the teacher gets out her stretchy frog and toad toys.

Max: The teacher asks Max, "Who should read the first page?" Max points to Patrick (Goal 1, maintenance skill). The teacher states, "Great, Patrick will read the first page," and hands the book to him.

Patrick: Patrick begins to read aloud but is speaking quickly, so the teacher puts her hand over the page and shows a card with the word *Slow* written on it. She then moves her hand and allows Patrick to continue reading (Goal 1). Patrick gets distracted by another student in the room and stops reading. The teacher holds the book in his line of sight and waits expectantly (Goal 3). Patrick reads one additional sentence, and the teacher allows him to choose one of the related stretchy toys. Another student begins to read aloud. After the student reads, "Why is that, Frog?" the teacher says, "Wait! Patrick, tell us what kind of sentence Toad said." Patrick replies, "A question sentence" (Goal 2). She tells Patrick, "That's right," and asks if he want a turn to read or wants to continue holding the stretchy toy. He chooses the toy.

Joy: The teacher then asks Joy, "What happened in the beginning of the story?" (Goals 1 and 3), and allows Joy to select who will read next after she answers the question. Joy chooses Max.

Max: The teacher asks Max, "What's our story about?" (Goals 1 and 3) Max answers, "Toad is sad," which is true but not the main plot of the story. The teacher decides to reinforce Max's attempt at answering because he made good eye contact. She models saying, "Frog and Toad are learning to fly a kite." She then hands Max the book to read aloud, which he enjoys.

The activity continues in this way, with everyone (including the teacher) taking turns reading aloud. The teacher provides stretchy toys to the students who have difficulty paying attention, so that they can remain with the group; she uses them to reinforce students' participation in the activity as well. Later these can be faded as students get better at staying in the group.

The student profile and group activity examples highlight how CPRT can be used across classroom curricula and with students of varied ability levels. Now that you have an idea of how IEP goals can be written and classroom activities organized with CPRT in mind, you can focus on teaching specific types of skills via CPRT. Communication skills, object play skills, social interaction skills, and academic skills are discussed in the next four sections.

Communication Skills

Where to Begin

As with all of the skills discussed in this chapter, you need to begin with each student's areas of strength and weakness. When you are deciding on specific goals for each student, a developmental assessment can be helpful. You can review the assessments done by the school psychologist or speech and language pathologist, and ask the parents to complete a communication checklist. You can also observe your student's communication skills in different settings. It is best to begin with communication skills your student is ready to learn, based on his developmental level. This helps to improve motivation and reduce failure. For example, if a 5-year-old student is at a 12-month level of communication development, CPRT acquisition goals may include sound imitation and early word imitation for highly familiar words, with maintenance tasks including babbling and reaching toward a preferred toy. Alternatively, a 10-year-old student with language skills at the 5-year level may be learning appropriate conversational skills, ways to ask and answer questions, and appropriate pronoun usage.

Topics of conversation and materials should be age-appropriate whenever possible. For example, a 10-year-old student can learn to talk about video games, sports, or music he enjoys, rather than only about toy trains or clay, even if the student may still find these "younger" toys interesting. This may help facilitate positive social interaction with the student's peers. However, a balance is important in order to capture the student's motivation.

When to Teach

Communication skills can be integrated into almost any activity throughout the school day. Therefore, with some planning, students can be required to use communication skills all day long. Make only small pieces of items available. Put preferred items up high. Even students who do *not* want to do something can communicate that by saying, "No, thank you," gesturing to move away from the table, or asking for a new activity. Communication, then, can be taught during one-on-one lessons, during small- or large-group activities, during snack time, on the playground, and even in the hallway. Always be on the lookout for ways to help your students use communication skills throughout each activity. Remember that communication is more than just words. Students can use gestures, sign language, pictures, and sounds to communicate their needs.

Students almost always need something, so you can "play dumb" and require your students to ask for what they need.

 More information about the development of communication skills can be found at *www.childdevelopmentinfo.com/development/language_development.shtml.*

How to Move Forward

Once your student has mastered the first step toward a particular goal, you can begin to require a more difficult response. However, it is always important to mix in some easy (maintenance) tasks to ensure that your student feels successful, and to reward your student when he makes a good effort, even if it is not perfect. One common issue when moving on to more complex communication skills is moving too quickly and asking a student to imitate skills beyond his developmental level, while not rewarding spontaneous communication at mastered levels. For example, a student may be able to use 10–20 single words spontaneously some of the time, so a teacher may move forward to have the student imitate two-word phrases. If the student is always required to use two-word phrases, and is not rewarded for spontaneous use of single words, the student is likely to stop communicating independently and will learn to wait for a prompt from the teacher. For students with autism, initiating spontaneous communication is often very difficult. Therefore, it is very important to continue to reward this student for simple, spontaneous initiations. There is a balance between expecting too much and not expecting enough. You will learn through experience how to push your students just enough to move them forward without having them become frustrated. *Table 5.4* contains IEP goals and curriculum areas, discussions of where to begin with students at various levels of communication, and information on how to move forward as students accomplish initial goals.

Object Play Skills

Where to Begin

CPRT has proven to be structured enough to help students learn simple to complex play skills, yet flexible enough to allow them to remain creative in their play. Research on play and autism has shown that children learn specific play skills more quickly when they are developmentally ready. So, again, assessment and observation of a student's skills will tell you where to begin.

Choose activities a student enjoys, and expect play skills at or just above the student's developmental level.

In addition, consider activities that are age-appropriate and/or ways to adapt activities that peers enjoy to meet each student's skill level. New activities and topics can be mixed with toys a student really likes, in order to encourage her to try new toys or actions. Toys that cross levels of play by providing opportunities for both cause-and-effect play and higher-level symbolic play can help increase play complexity when CPRT is used. For example, a fire station that makes authentic noises can be used to pretend to fight a fire.

When you are teaching play skills using CPRT, use the same steps you would use when facilitating communication skills. Instead of expecting your student to gesture or talk to obtain an item, you will expect her to complete a play action. CPRT can be used to teach a range of play skills from early manipulative play through sociodramatic play (see *Table 5.5* for a list of play skill stages).

 Use *Handout 2: Object Play Level Progression* in *Part IV* to assess your student's current level of play skills.

TABLE 5.4. Communication Skills

This table provides sample goals and ideas of where to begin and how to move forward with teaching communication skills using CPRT.

Sample annual IEP goal or curriculum area	Where to begin	How to move forward
Joey will use early communication strategies (such as reaching, pointing, or making a purposeful vocalization) to obtain desired items during 8 of 10 opportunities in a small-group setting.	Require early communication skills before giving the student access to the item. Joey is learning that his actions and vocalizations can be communicative, so use a high number of maintenance tasks and reinforce attempts at a high rate until he clearly understands the connection between his actions and the reinforcer.	Once Joey clearly understands the connection between his actions and accessing reinforcement (e.g., an object or an activity with you or a peer), you can require vocalizations more often, and begin to shape these vocalizations to be closer to words, while continuing to reward gestures at least 50% of the time.
Marta will use five new initial word sounds—/b/, /m/, /o/, /e/, and /l/—to request preferred items beginning with those specific sounds (e.g., /b/ for *ball*) in 80% of opportunities.	Begin with sounds Marta is able to say easily, and reward those sounds with the appropriate items. Then shape her sounds by using reinforcement of attempts to move her closer and closer to the appropriate sound.	When Marta has learned to make each sound, begin to require that sound (or a good approximation) for each item she wants. You can begin to require a few trials before rewarding an attempt, in order to shape the correct sound.
Saul will obtain the attention of the listener by using an appropriate strategy (e.g., tapping on and/or calling that person's name, then waiting for an appropriate response) in 8 of 10 trials in the classroom.	Begin by lifting Saul's hand to help him tap you and gain attention before having him use communication skills to request or comment.	After Saul is consistently tapping to gain attention, wait a few seconds before responding. You can have him look toward you while communicating or calling your name before requesting, to make the skill more complex.
Julia will learn to label 5–10 new words per month, and will use these new words in at least 2 settings with at least 2 different adults and/or peers.	Ensure that favored items are available in several settings. Be sure to have several examples of each item (several cars, different types of markers, etc.). Require Julia to use the label to access these items in the different settings. Be sure that different adults and peers expect this level of communication throughout the day.	Make this more complex by using new examples of items Julia has mastered, by having her label novel items she may not see on a daily basis, and by using expectant waiting to encourage spontaneous use of the words she has mastered. For example, use different colors and sizes of blocks, and different types of vehicles or new animals.

(cont.)

TABLE 5.4. *(cont.)*

Sample annual IEP goal or curriculum area	Where to begin	How to move forward
Peter will answer yes–no questions to indicate his needs and wants (e.g., "Do you want to jump?"), when given 1 visual cue (e.g., gesture, picture symbol), during 80% of opportunities.	Ask yes–no questions multiple times throughout the day. If you know the correct answer (e.g., you know that Peter does not like pickles), prompt the appropriate response using a known gesture or picture card and the appropriate facial expression (e.g., wrinkled nose). Remember, if he answers incorrectly, be sure to offer or withhold the item based on Peter's response so that he will learn the natural consequence of his communication.	As Peter masters this skill, reduce your prompts—first from picture to gesture, then to an expectant look—and, finally, expect a spontaneous response.
Amir will produce 3- to 5-word phrases for a variety of communicative purposes (e.g., to request, label, greet), across 3 activities (e.g., circle time, structured play), given 1 verbal or visual cue, on 5 of 5 school days.	When Amir is requesting an item or commenting, wait for a 3- to 5-word phrase at least half the time. At first, these longer phrases will need to be prompted using a verbal or gestural cue. Be sure to reward attempts (1- to 2-word phrases) and to intersperse maintenance tasks to keep motivation high.	Again, reduce your cues as Amir masters the use of phrase speech. Be sure to vary phrases, and use meaningful words to reduce stereotyped responding—for example, "Pass the red apple" instead of "I want apple, please."
Mei Lein will communicate how she is feeling and how others are feeling, and explain why, on 4 of 5 opportunities over 5 days.	Begin with one feeling that is easy to identify (e.g., happy or sad). Have Mei Lein identify this feeling in other people, or in photos. Add new feelings as she masters each feeling in others and in books.	Once Mei Lein can identify obvious feelings in others, have her model feelings for you, and identify them in herself. Begin to identify her feelings with her and help her explain why (only if you know). Try to use a book, doll, or activity where she can describe emotions and receive the item as a reinforcer. For example, ask her to "Show me how the mouse feels in the story when it sees the cat," and then allow her to look at the pictures in the book as she likes when she answers or attempts to answer the question correctly.
Caroline will retell a familiar story to include a character, problem, and resolution after listening to or reading a literary text on 2 consecutive occasions.	Begin by reading a page of a story together and having Caroline retell the main points of the story. Moving on with a preferred story can be contingent upon her talking about the pictures or topic on the page.	Gradually increase the length of the story Caroline needs to listen to or read before retelling the story. Move on to more novel stories as she becomes better at this skill. Be sure to allow her to choose the story or topic to increase motivation.

TABLE 5.5. Play Levels and Examples

In addition to listing play levels in increasing order of complexity, this table provides a variety of toys that may be useful in targeting specific types of play.

Types of play	Examples	Toy ideas
Manipulative play	• Dumping toys out • Putting toys in • Operational toys • Construction play (blocks) • Puzzles • Rough-and-tumble play	• Noisy toys • Toys with lights • Spinning toys • Cars that go down ramps • Koosh balls • Bubbles • Puzzles • Tactile materials (e.g., sand, beads, shaving cream, clay)
Representational play	• Pretend play toward self (e.g., brushing own hair) • Events that happen daily • Single activities • Realistic props • Pretend play toward self and other people (same action), then beginning to pretend toward doll • Caregiver activities • Combining two toys or performing actions on two people	• Garage with cars • Play food/pots and pans, etc. • Doctor kit • Doll house • Toys with dolls, as well as with manipulative parts that are fun (e.g., doors to open, ramps to roll things down)
Symbolic play	• Talking to doll • Events personally experienced that happen periodically; emotions • Several actions on a theme (doll in tub, wash, dry) • Beginning to use object substitutions • Giving voice to dolls • Events child has seen or heard about but not personally experienced • Short sequences of time-related activities • Less realistic props • Dolls taking action • Events evolving • Giving characters multiple roles • Planned events with cause–effect sequences	• Representational toys • Any representational toys plus "junk" • Boxes • String • Sponges • Movie character figures • Tea sets, etc. • Blocks
Sociodramatic play	• Highly imaginative themes • Pretending to have a role and "be" a character • Multiple planned sequences • Familiar and novel fantasy themes	• Symbolic play materials • Dress-up clothes • Firefighter equipment • Doctor kit • Baby dolls with food, bed, stroller, etc. • Lots of functional toys (food, cash register, etc.) • Household items

(cont.)

TABLE 5.5. *(cont.)*		
Types of play	**Examples**	**Toy ideas**
Games with rules	• Simple board games involving chance only • Games that require chance and skill • Skill-based games • Cooperative games requiring team play and score keeping	• Chutes and Ladders • Candyland • Crocodile Dentist • Ants in the Pants • Don't Break the Ice • Games with movie characters the child enjoys • Organized sports

Using the specific steps of CPRT to teach symbolic play may begin with a student choosing to play with a set of toy cars (choice). The student typically plays functionally with the toy cars, completing actions like washing the car, filling it with gas, or parking it. You give the student a block and ask, "What can we do with these toys?" (acquisition). The student is expected to use the block symbolically—for example, as a sponge to "wash" the car. If the student does not respond, you can model the symbolic behavior (turn taking) along with appropriate language: "Wash the car." You then return the block to the student. If the student does not respond but is still interested in the cars, you can provide a direct instruction to wash the car, and/or use gestural or hand-over-hand assistance to ensure the student's success. When the student does respond (either on his own or with some help), give him the entire set of cars to play with in any manner he chooses (contingent, direct reinforcement of the new behavior). This may include using the toy in a stereotyped manner. You have the opportunity to model more complex play and provide new play ideas on your turn.

Just as when you are teaching communication skills, the play skill level to target will depend on the student. One student may be learning to complete a puzzle or draw on paper, while another student may be learning to pretend to pack the car for a trip to the zoo where she pretends to see animals and perhaps have a picnic. Students can learn games with rules, large motor games, and fine motor play using CPRT. As with communication, typically developing children do not completely abandon simpler forms of play as they gain new skills. In order to keep play natural, you will want to combine various levels of play. This makes it easy to use both maintenance and acquisition tasks while teaching play.

When to Teach

Making time for play during the school day is very important for individuals with autism because even those who are academically gifted continue to have difficulty with social interaction and leisure skills throughout their lives. Play skills can be taught at recess, at lunch, and during snack time. In addition, there may be a specified choice or play time in the classroom between academic activities, at arrival, or before dismissal, when these vital play skills can be addressed. Regardless of when they are taught, skills learned during play activities should generalize to other parts of the school day. For example, learning to sequence play actions is correlated with putting phrases together.

It is important to make time for practicing play, as this will also increase communication and other aspects of each student's development.

Play skills help children practice turn taking and problem solving.

How to Move Forward

Again, once your student has mastered the first step toward a particular goal, you can begin to require a more difficult response. It is still important to mix in some easy (maintenance) tasks to ensure that your student feels successful, and to reward your student for good trying. Even though play is fun for most kids, it can be a difficult skill for students with autism; otherwise, we wouldn't need to teach it! As noted above, play skills follow a developmental progression; begin your teaching at the developmental level appropriate for your student. Once your student has mastered that level with a variety of materials in several settings and is beginning to use that play skill independently, it is time to move to the next play stage. This may involve moving from pushing buttons on a busy box to building with blocks, or from one-step symbolic play actions to two-step schemes. Students will need to move between different play levels as they learn to play spontaneously. Remember, make it fun! You are playing, after all. *Table 5.6* contains IEP goals and curriculum areas, discussions of where to begin with students at various levels of play skills, and information on how to move forward as students accomplish initial goals.

Social Interaction Skills
Where to Begin

In teaching social skills to students with autism, it is especially important to begin with early foundational skills. Students with autism may have cognitive and communicative skills that are more advanced than their ability to understand and participate in social interactions. Social interactions are very complex, and individual skills tend to build upon each other; therefore, it is very important to teach the basic skills that are the building blocks for later, more sophisticated interactions. Again, CPRT has been proven to be useful for increasing a variety of social skills in children with autism, including early joint attention skills, responding to peer initiations, and initiating with both peers and adults.

- Looking when someone points to an object nearby.
- Looking when someone points to an object far away.
- Looking when someone looks at something interesting across the room.
- Showing items or others (e.g., holding up a toy or completed work for someone to see).
- Pointing to something interesting nearby.
- Pointing to something interesting far away.

All of these require sharing attention with the partner.

FIGURE 5.1. Stages of Joint Attention. Students with autism often have difficulty sharing attention with a partner. It may be necessary to specifically teach the earlier stages of joint attention to some students, to help them move forward in this area.

See *Chapter 9* for a description of the research supporting CPRT as an effective method for teaching social skills.

TABLE 5.6. Object Play Skills

This table provides sample goals and ideas of where to begin and how to move forward with teaching object play skills using CPRT.

Sample IEP annual goal or curriculum area	Where to begin	How to move forward
Joey will engage in simple manipulative play with blocks, gears, puzzles, or balls independently for a period of 10 minutes during play time in the classroom.	Require early manipulative skills before giving Joey access to the item. Begin by gaining Joey's attention as he plays with blocks. Take a turn and complete a new action with the block (put in a cup; stack). Help Joey put a block in the cup (a new action for him). Reinforce Joey by allowing him to play with the blocks in any way he chooses.	Increase the amount of time Joey is required to play appropriately with the toy before allowing independent play. Begin to introduce new play activities. Combine activities Joey has mastered and enjoys with new activities at first, in order to reward Joey and help him become familiar with new toys.
Marta will sit at a table in a small group and manually manipulate varied materials (e.g., play clay shaving cream, sand) for a period of 5 minutes independently.	Begin by finding materials Marta enjoys and making them available alongside the less desired materials. For example, if Marta loves balls, begin by having her roll a ball in play clay to gain free access to the ball. Be sure to take turns modeling appropriate behavior, and make it look fun! Reinforce Marta with free access to the ball.	As Marta becomes comfortable with each material, increase her exposure to it. For example, put her favorite toy deep in the sand for her to dig out rather than having her roll it on top of the sand. Increase slowly and intersperse maintenance tasks regularly.
Saul will engage in 2-step play actions with cars and trains with moderate support for a 10-minute period during recess.	Saul tends to line up cars and trains instead of using them playfully. Begin by using modeling (turn taking), verbal instructions, and hand-over-hand assistance to help Saul roll cars down a ramp or into a garage, or move trains around a track. Once he completes one step, he can be rewarded with free access to the toys and be allowed to line the toys up for a short period before trying again.	Once Saul has begun to do single-step actions independently and/or spontaneously, begin to require 2-step actions before allowing Saul free access to the cars or trains. Be sure to take turns and model new 2-step actions. Also, be sure to vary the actions you put together and require from Saul, so that his play does not become stereotyped. Extend the time he will play on his own through turn taking and extending the time before he is rewarded.
Julia will learn to perform 5 new representational play actions per month, and will use these new actions in a sequence of at least 3 steps.	Julia enjoys playing with dolls, but primarily carries them around. She is able to pretend to talk on the phone on her own. Begin by expecting Julia to complete one new action at a time with the doll (e.g., feeding the doll with a spoon) before allowing her free access to the doll. Choose 1–3 actions to work on with support until Julia is able to complete these independently. Join her in play to make it more natural and to allow modeling of new play actions and turn taking.	Once Julia can use 1–3 actions independently, it is time to move on as described in the examples above. Again, make your play as natural as possible, expecting different types of actions and more difficult tasks (such as having dolls "act" or the baby doll "cry"), to encourage more symbolic play.

(cont.)

TABLE 5.6. *(cont.)*

Sample IEP annual goal or curriculum area	Where to begin	How to move forward
Peter will play appropriately on the playground using play equipment, sand toys, and balls for at least 80% of recess.	Peter enjoys being outside, but often engages in self-stimulatory behavior. He tends to pick grass and sift sand. Begin using activities Peter enjoys, such as sand play. Require Peter to dig in the sand several times with a shovel before being rewarded with sifting. Allow Peter to roll a ball to his friend through the sand. Have his friend take a turn with the ball by rolling it back. Have Peter scoot a bike on the grass, then back to the path, and reward him with going back to the grass. Increase the time required to get to reinforcement. You could also integrate other strategies with CPRT, such as use of a picture schedule to help Peter navigate through various play activities during time on the playground.	Continue to increase the time Peter needs to play appropriately before allowing him to play on his own or engage in self-stimulatory behavior. Again, be creative in including Peter's favorite activities with new ones. As he becomes familiar with the new activities, he is likely to begin to engage in those on his own, and his self-stimulatory behaviors may begin to decrease as a result.
Amir will participate in an organized game of kickball with his classmates with minimal support, and will remain engaged for at least 80% of the game.	Amir has difficulty remaining engaged during organized games. He enjoys throwing and kicking the ball, but does not like to run. Allow Amir to choose the color of the ball he would like to kick. Begin by requiring Amir to run to home base before he is allowed to kick the ball. Do this one-on-one or in a small group at first, before having Amir try a real game. Add more bases as he gets better at running, rewarding him with throwing the ball (even if it is not in the rule book). Once he is ready to try a real game, you can combine strategies and use some external praise or reinforcement if changing the game is upsetting to other students. Allow Amir to hold a ball as long as he is engaging in the game. In the outfield, place him in a position that requires throwing the ball.	In the best of all possible worlds, Amir will begin to enjoy kickball as he becomes familiar with the game. This is most likely to be the case if he is developmentally ready to learn to play a team sport. Expand the amount of time he is engaged before gaining reinforcement. Be creative in finding direct reinforcement that makes him intrinsically motivated to play the game. Perhaps he enjoys numbers and can count the number of outs or how many players get to kick, for example.
Mei Lein will complete a board game, taking turns and following the rules of the game independently.	Allow Mei Lein to choose a game she enjoys, or find a game that includes a character she likes. Think about the aspects of the game that Mei Lein may like: putting pieces on the board, counting the spaces, rolling the dice, labeling colors, etc. Creatively find a way to reward Mei Lein for playing the game correctly with another aspect of the game she enjoys. You might incorporate a figure or picture of her favorite character as a game piece, for example. Starting with games that are manipulative, such as Don't Break the Ice or Ants in the Pants, can help increase interest. Show her how the game is really played when it is your turn.	As Mei Lein becomes proficient with new games, try to fade the presence of her favored characters and replace them with the original game pieces. This can be done when she begins to enjoy the game itself. Increase the number of turns she needs to take before gaining access to her reinforcer. Incorporate fun activities as part of some games, for example, if Mei Lein enjoys drawing, perhaps she can draw with a pen of the same color as the square she lands on when playing Sorry; or you can add some real candy to certain squares on the Candyland game. When direct reinforcers are incorporated, Mei Lein will be more likely to begin to enjoy the game as those rewards and supports are faded.

(cont.)

TABLE 5.6. *(cont.)*

Sample IEP annual goal or curriculum area	Where to begin	How to move forward
Caroline will engage in sociodramatic play schemes of 10–20 steps while playing with a peer in the classroom.	Begin by having Caroline choose an activity or topic for her play—for example, going to the zoo, playing house, playing doctor, or going on a train ride. Incorporate some objects she likes (perhaps animals, dolls, cars). Caroline can earn access to the objects or topics she enjoys by engaging in several steps of sociodramatic play. For example, have Caroline pretend to set up a bus with her friend, and together they can ride to the zoo, pretend to feed some animals (and get rewarded with play with toy animals), then clean some cages, see an animal show (play with more toy animals), have cotton candy, get back on the bus, and drive home. Allow her friend to model new ways to play during her turn.	When Caroline is allowed to choose play activities and to incorporate favorite toys into play, she should enjoy this play, even though it is difficult. You will be using maintenance tasks and rewarding attempts to keep her motivated and engaged. Of course, her peers may wish to choose activities as well, so as Caroline gets better at pretending, she can allow her friends a turn at choosing the game. A more difficult task for her will be to actually pretend to be another person (e.g., a firefighter), rather than simply doing pretend activities as herself.

Let's begin by examining the procedures used to teach joint attention skills. Engaging in **joint attention** means sharing an experience with someone else by looking, pointing, or gesturing and making sure that the other person is also looking. *Figure 5.1* (on page 86) highlights the stages of joint attention. This skill is essential for learning, and it is often lacking or delayed in students with autism. The first stage of joint attention involves responding to others' bids for attention. This includes showing the student a toy or a poster, or drawing his attention to the whiteboard. To teach this skill, you should begin by using objects that are near the student and incorporating gestures or words toward which the student is to direct his attention. For all instruction on joint attention, use items that you know will interest the student.

To teach a student with autism to look to a new object that someone else is attending to (responding to joint attention), follow this process:

1. *Shifting attention.* Place the student's hand on a new item when she is engaged with something else (e.g., a pen of different color when she is using a crayon). Reward the student for paying attention to and engaging with the new item by providing free access to both items (either the new item or the one she already has, depending on which she wants). Gradually fade the level of prompting from placing the student's hand on the object, to tapping the object, to showing the student the object by simply holding it out.

2. *Adding eye contact.* Once the student is easily shifting attention to the new object, begin to make the response more complex by expecting the student to make eye contact with you before rewarding the behavior.

3. *Gaining attention with eye contact.* Once eye contact is occurring regularly, gain the student's attention with your own eye contact and expect her to follow a point to a new object. Begin close to the new object, and gradually expect the student to follow a point to objects that are farther away. Next, move to pointing to pic-

tures and other items of interest around the room, reinforcing the child with continued access to the current object or discussion of the interesting item you are pointing out (perhaps one of her favorite movies or some of her peers).

Following these steps, you can systematically teach your student to respond to joint attention bids. This skill will be an important building block for further learning because it helps the student gather information from watching others and leads to an increase in imitation skills.

Initiating joint attention can be much more difficult to teach. This skill requires intrinsic motivation to want to share information simply to be social. Often students with autism are not motivated to share information or accomplishments with others in the same way that other students do. For example, your student may be less likely to show you a picture he drew or to point out a hot-air balloon flying over the playground. Reinforcing joint attention initiation is also a challenge because you need to be sure to distinguish commenting and sharing from requesting. When a student makes a request by looking at something or pointing, the reward is receiving the item. However, if a student is using the same behaviors to share an experience (initiate joint attention), the reward is your attention alone. This means that if a student points out something "cool" for you to look at (e.g., a picture on the wall), you shouldn't hand him the picture because that is no longer sharing information; it has become requesting. Instead, the reward needs to be your attention. This is an area where it may be helpful to integrate more general ABA-based strategies, such as the use of indirect reinforcers. However, if natural reinforcers can be used, this will increase generalization of skills.

It is important that you set up opportunities specifically for teaching initiating joint attention so your students learn how their behavior can lead to different positive consequences.

To teach a student with autism to share something interesting in the environment with someone else (initiating joint attention), follow this process:

1. *Showing when asked.* Begin by asking the student to show you or a peer objects, work she is doing, and other items of interest. Be sure that she is also shifting her eye gaze to the person to whom she is showing the item. Again, you can begin with verbal prompts or physical prompts (helping the student hold the item up to show someone), and fade your help until the student can show the item on her own.

2. *Pointing to indicate interest.* The next step is to teach your student to point to interesting things in the environment simply to share information (this is known as protodeclarative pointing). To support this step, it is helpful to have some new, interesting items or pictures in the classroom that your student will notice and enjoy talking about. Again, verbal or physical prompts to point can be used at first and then faded. If you do this activity when your student is doing something she enjoys, she can continue with the activity as a reinforcer. Generalize these new skills by practicing in different areas of the classroom and school campus, as well as on field trips.

3. *Pairing pointing with eye contact.* The final step is to require your student to make eye contact while sharing attention. It may be helpful to move into

your student's line of sight after she has pointed to something to facilitate this eye contact, and then slowly fade this prompt as your student becomes more proficient at shifting her eye contact to you after pointing.

Once your students have a foundation in joint attention, you can move to teaching increasingly complex social skills. *Figure 5.2* lists the stages of social interaction. More advanced social interaction skills can be rewarded naturally. For example, when a student asks to take a turn, he gets to engage in the activity he desires. When a student is learning to give a turn, others' turns should be brief, and the student should get to take his next turn without having to make an additional response (he is rewarded for waiting while the other person took a turn). Passing out snacks to peers and asking what they want can be rewarded with getting to choose a snack or preferred item. For some students, simply being allowed to have a role as a helper is reinforcing, so they can continue to help as long as they continue to complete the task as they are supposed to do.

- Solitary: Plays alone with little interaction.
- Spectator: Observes other students, but does not play with them.
- Parallel: Plays alongside others, but not together.
- Associate: Starts to interact with others in play with brief cooperation. Friendships begin to develop.
- Cooperative: Plays together with shared goals of others. Can be supportive of other students during play. Understands games with rules.

FIGURE 5.2. **Stages of Social Interaction.** Students move from solitary to cooperative play as they develop.

When to Teach

The specific time to teach social interaction skills will vary, depending on the skill being taught. For example, joint attention can be taught throughout the day when a student has an opportunity to show you a completed worksheet, a favorite toy, or a tractor outside the window. Playing dolls with a peer is likely to happen during a structured play time. Practicing conversation skills can occur during circle time, during a discussion of state capitals, or at lunch time. Even simple interactions can be difficult for students with autism, so having a student collect worksheets or pass out pencils can help her practice social skills. A reward for correctly completing these activities could be choosing a special pencil or counting the completed worksheets. Your student may complete these tasks differently, depending upon her developmental level. For example, one student may need you to give him each pencil and point to the student she needs to hand it to. A more verbal student may have a bunch of pencils and be able to ask each peer to choose a color.

How to Move Forward

Social skills are likely to be the most difficult skills you will work on for many students with autism. It may also seem more difficult for them to use these skills naturally. As you move forward, observe each student using new social skills. If a student does not interact naturally, or if his behavior does not generalize to new people and situations, work on spontaneity and flexibility before moving forward too quickly. Be intentional in the way you use social interaction with your student, keeping your voice natural and using different prompts and responses. For example, when students ask each other for a turn, they may use various methods: saying, "My turn," reaching out an open hand, saying, "Give it to me," asking, "Can I try?", or asking for the object by name. Students who are learning to maintain conversations can practice talking about their favorite topic in a variety of ways. Observe other students of the same age who do not have social impairments, to get ideas for appropriate and varied ways to interact. *Table 5.7* contains IEP goals and curriculum areas, discussions of where to begin with students at various levels of social interaction skills, and information on how to move forward as students accomplish initial goals.

Because social interactions are complex and confusing, you may find that students make slower progress on social goals than goals in other areas.

Academic Skills

Where to Begin

Teaching academic skills using CPRT may require some creativity and minor modification to your usual lessons. Some components of CPRT are easy to incorporate into academic tasks, such as gaining your students' attention and providing clear and appropriate cues. Other components may require you to adapt lessons and be creative with materials. Using student choice, turn taking, multiple cues, and direct reinforcement, for example, are not always considered when academic tasks are taught. As with any new skill set, begin with an assessment of the student's current skill level in the curriculum area. What are the student's math, reading, and writing skills? Use your state standards and/or school curriculum to determine the appropriate starting place and progression in each specific area.

Although CPRT may not be the right strategy for all academic tasks, it can be effectively used to increase motivation and learning in many cases.

The first challenge in teaching academic skills is providing students with a choice to enhance motivation. One simple way is to have more than one option available. For example, you may allow your student to choose which worksheet to complete, what book/topic to read, or where to sit (e.g., at the table or in the quiet area). Students working in a group can also make choices as to what section they would like to read, what color marker they would like to use to write on the board, and so forth. You can also provide various colors and types of writing utensils to target multiple cues within writing tasks. Including topics the students enjoy or using stickers of preferred characters can help make academic learning more fun. For instance, Mickey Mouse can travel through Europe to help teach the students about geography. Again, be creative! In the case of academics, choices may be more limited than when you are working on play or social skills. However, you can follow students' leads and still meet your teaching goals. For example, one student may bring up French toast during the geography lesson, which could lead to some research about how the name was developed. You can incorporate students' specialized interests, such as dolphins, by mapping where dolphins live and routes used for migration. Students may be allowed to work together to develop the daily schedule or to choose when to do math versus English. The main focus should be on maximizing student motivation by targeting individual students' interests and by sharing control of the learning environment.

TABLE 5.7. Social Interaction Skills

This table provides sample goals and ideas of where to begin and how to move forward with teaching social interaction skills using CPRT.

Sample IEP annual goal or curriculum area	Where to begin	How to move forward
Joey will remain in proximity to peers (within 2 feet) during small-group activities in the classroom and on the playground for at least 10 minutes with minimal prompting.	Begin by prompting students to remain in a group setting. Start with very brief periods of time at circle time, at the table, and during play time, where Joey needs to remain near his peers. Reward Joey by allowing him to continue to engage in a preferred activity. Being fun can help ensure that students will group together. For example, if Joey loves bubbles, blow bubbles on the playground in a way that encourages other students to come and play as well.	Once Joey is able to tolerate brief periods of time around other children, increase the time Joey is expected to remain in the group. You can also begin to increase the size of the group. Continue to have activities Joey enjoys in the group setting. Once he is successfully staying in the group with favored activities, periods of time sitting and listening or doing other activities can be rewarded with access to his favorite things.
Marta will engage in a chasing/fleeing game with peers for 5 minutes, with physical and verbal prompts as needed, on 4 of 5 opportunities at recess.	Gross motor/chase games are often fun for children with autism and offer a good place to start peer interaction. Require Marta to tap her peer and run a short way, and prompt the peer to chase her (Marta's reward). Next, have the peer tap Marta and prompt Marta to chase the peer. This may be enjoyable in and of itself, or the peer may have an item Marta likes that she can access by playing chase.	Often as students learn to play games, the game itself becomes reinforcing. Reduce your prompts for Marta and see if she will begin to play chase on her own. If she enjoys the game, you can teach her a more structured game of tag and reduce your prompting even further.
Saul will engage in reciprocal play activities with one or two familiar peers, by saying "Hi," requesting "My turn," and requesting objects, with adult facilitation on 4 of 5 opportunities.	Begin by finding materials Saul enjoys and having peers engage with those same materials (e.g., cars and trains). Prompt Saul to wave or say "Hi" when he joins the group, and to request "My turn" or ask for an object. Since using language along with social interaction may be difficult for Saul, he can use a gesture or picture to indicate that he wants a turn. He can learn to trade toys at first if turn taking is difficult.	Once Saul is trading toys and taking turns, you can increase the length of his peers' turns. Peers can provide play suggestions for Saul to follow before he gains free access to his preferred toy. Incorporating new toys with cars and trucks can help Saul learn to enjoy other toys that his peers may be interested in.
Given minimal (1–2) prompts, Julia will participate with a familiar peer in a familiar/rehearsed pretend theme play, using theme-appropriate language to comment, request, and negotiate, on 4 of 5 opportunities during the school week.	Since Julia is working on increasing her play actions on her own, she can also work on doing this with her peers. Expect Julie to play with her dolls with peers. Require her to feed her peer's doll or allow a peer to give her doll a drink. Reward Julie with free access to the toys. Encourage the students to ask each other if it is okay to feed the other doll. Help them generate ideas of what to do next, while still maximizing their independent play.	Increase the number of actions Julia will allow her peer to do, or the number of exchanges she needs to complete, before she gains free access to the toys. In addition, require her to talk about what she wants to do next and/or ask her play partner what she would like to do next. Language, play, and social interaction goals are relevant in this play scenario and can be targeted simultaneously.

(cont.)

TABLE 5.7. *(cont.)*

Sample IEP annual goal or curriculum area	Where to begin	How to move forward
Peter will maintain an appropriate distance for personal space while interacting with peers in 8 of 10 opportunities.	Begin by commenting on the distance a person should maintain as personal space while interacting with Peter. Allow Peter to talk about his preferred topic, as long as he does not come too close.	Once Peter is successfully monitoring his personal space while interacting with you and other adults, encourage him to practice with peers. Provide a subtle gestural prompt to remind him to maintain distance when necessary. Peter is motivated by interacting with his peers; briefly remove him from the interaction if he fails to maintain an appropriate distance.
Amir will participate in an organized game that requires peer interaction for at least 4–5 exchanges independently.	Since we know that Amir likes to throw and catch, begin by having him play catch with a peer. The reward is built into the game. As long as Amir plays catch with his friend, he can continue to throw and catch the ball.	As Amir gets better at staying with his peer, add additional peers or complexity. Play Four Square for a few minutes and then go back to catch.
Mei Lein will independently use and respond to questions, comments, and directives to maintain a conversation over several turns (3–5) with peers, while using appropriate eye contact, during varied play and classroom activities on 4 of 5 occasions over 3 consecutive trial days.	Allow Mei Lein to choose a game or topic she enjoys. If there are topics or games that overlap with what other students in the class enjoy, it may be best to start working on this goal with those students. Assist Mei Lein with verbal and visual prompts to maintain a conversation for a few turns, ensuring that she has appropriate eye contact during the conversation. She may need help asking questions or waiting for the other student to comment. She can be rewarded by using materials as she wishes or simply by continuing to get to talk about her favorite topic. If she does not use good eye contact, you can change the topic of conversation until she makes a good attempt or is successful.	Gradually increase the number of exchanges Mei Lein is required to have before she can access her favorite toy or continue with her topic. Eventually, you can introduce short periods of time when she is talking about a topic suggested by her peer.
Caroline will use 5- to 10-word sentences when responding to adults and peers, and ask questions or make appropriate comments to maintain conversation while staying on topic, for at least 5 minutes on 4 of 5 opportunities over 5 days.	Begin by having Caroline choose an activity or topic for her play—for example, her recent trip to the zoo, her pet cat, or a movie she likes. Caroline can earn access to related toys (animals), or may continue to talk about her favorite topic, by maintaining conversation with her partner. For example, have Caroline tell a friend what silly thing her cat did this weekend. She must then ask her friend if she has any pets (she may need a prompt to do this in the beginning). She is required to comment appropriately on her friend's statement ("Oh, you have a dog? I like dogs"), and she can then go back to talking about her cat ("My cat likes milk").	Gradually increase the number of varied topics that Caroline will discuss. This can be done by integrating new topics with her favorite topics. For example, you can introduce the topic of swimming. Caroline can discuss whether or not her cat might like to swim, and ask a peer whether or not he likes to swim, where he swims, etc. Again, reward her with access to her favorite topics. Ideally, peer attention will become rewarding as time goes on. If your attention is rewarding to Caroline, you can participate in the conversation when she is successful or trying hard.

Review the *Component 4: Shared Control* section of *Chapter 4* for tips on how to provide choices within a group.

 Reserving highly preferred materials for use with less preferred activities or lessons is a good way to incorporate direct reinforcement into academic tasks.

Another special challenge in working on academic tasks can be finding direct reinforcers. What is the direct reinforcer for completing a math problem? This will depend on the student. One student may find highlighting each completed math problem reinforcing (especially if he only has access to highlighter pens during math time). Another student may choose to count beads that correspond with the answers to each problem. Yet another student may simply enjoy getting to the next activity (which may be choosing a book or going outside) upon careful completion of the assignment. Sometimes task completion can be reinforcing on its own. For example, when the task is matching sight words with corresponding pictures, finding the correct pairs can be rewarding for some students. Others may enjoy the competitiveness of gathering the most correct answers in a group, or racing to beat a timer you have set. Some students may enjoy putting the completed sets in a "mailbox." Students working on handwriting can trace or write their requests for certain objects in order to access them (e.g., writing "Fill the yellow cup with milk and pass it to me"). Drawers can be labeled with sight words for students to read before getting the item. These are just a few ideas to get you started. Brainstorm with other adults in your classroom, and identify the best ways to use direct reinforcement with your students. Remember, reinforcement should always be based on student responses and should be related to the task.

Be sure to monitor each student's response in group situations. If students are working independently at their desks, check on their progress. Redirect students who are having difficulty or whose attention to the task is waning. It may be necessary to reward partial completion of tasks or provide choices within the activity, such as which questions to complete first. Turn taking and modeling appropriate answers can be helpful with teaching as well as rewarding to a student. Rewarding attempts remains an important way to keep motivation high.

 Take a few moments to take some notes about the best ways to use direct reinforcement with your students.

When to Teach

CPRT can be used any time you are teaching academics in either group or individual settings. Fun activities, such as cooking, can be used to teach measurement, sequencing, and reading sight words using CPRT. Less exciting tasks can be made more motivating by including topics or items that interest students. If you choose to teach a specific academic skill using other strategies, CPRT can still be very useful for helping to make the newly learned information useful and functional for your students, and to help with generalization of skills to other areas.

How to Move Forward

When to move forward may be easier to determine with academic skills than with more abstract skills. For example, once Mei Lein has learned to write single words accurately on her own, it is time to move on to having her write two- or three-word sentences. It is important that the newly learned skill be one the student can do independently and across a variety of materials and environments before you consider the skill to be mastered. Caroline may know how to identify North, South, East, and West in the classroom, but she also needs to be able to do so on a variety of maps, on the playground, at home, and in the community. In the case of academic skills, use the guidelines that your school follows for each grade level in each area. Don't forget to help your students remember the foundation skills for each annual goal by mixing in easy skills with the more difficult ones they are still learning. This will help with motivation as well as long-term use of skills. *Table 5.8* contains IEP goals and curriculum areas, discussions of where to begin with students targeting various academic skills, and information on how to move forward as students accomplish initial goals.

Chapter Summary

CPRT can be used to target the specific IEP and curriculum area goals of the students in your classroom. CPRT can be used to address the varying skill levels of different students during the same group activity, and the strategies can help keep children motivated and engaged while learning. Communication, play, social, and academic skills can all be targeted during a variety of group activities using CPRT strategies. Remember to base the instruction on the students' goals and developmental level, and to include time for play and social skills, as these will provide the basis for learning in other areas. CPRT strategies are flexible and can be used with any school-based curricula or state guidelines to meet the varied goals of the students in your classroom.

TABLE 5.8. Academic Skills

This table provides sample goals and ideas of where to begin and how to move forward with teaching academic skills using CPRT.

Sample annual IEP goal or curriculum area	Where to begin	How to move forward
With a verbal cue, Joey will match 5 objects (then pictures, colors, shapes) in a field of 3 with 90% accuracy over 2 trial days.	Begin with objects that Joey enjoys. Depending on his skill level, you can begin with identical items. Later, use multiple examples of various objects (e.g., several different types of cups with juice or milk) to enhance generalization. Start with one cup, and have Joey match it to pair with a field of just one. He gets the cup with juice as his reward. Increase the difficulty as he is ready. You can then also use nonpreferred objects in the task, putting the preferred object in the "field of 3" first. Require Joey to match, then allow him to choose the item he would like to play with, based on his correct response. Remember to take turns matching and to model appropriate play.	Once Joey is matching objects consistently, you can move to pictures, using the same strategy. The only difference is that Joey can trade the picture he has matched for the object he enjoys. Matching colors can be done in the context of other activities. For example, he can match colored pens to colored paper before getting to choose what to draw. He can match colored blocks (or blocks of different shapes) before gaining free access to the materials. If he wants to play with toy cars, he can sort the cars by color or type as he gets closer to mastering this goal.
Marta will copy a vertical and horizontal line, a circle, and a square accurately during 80% of opportunities.	If Marta enjoys drawing or using markers, allow her to choose the color of the marker, and reward her with free drawing. However, if she doesn't like to draw, you may need to build the drawing into another activity. Perhaps she needs to underline or circle the snack item she wants to eat or the song she wants to sing. If she is motivated by peer interaction, have her imitate a peer's drawing in order to get to join in a drawing game. If she likes to count, she can draw a line to connect numbers. Begin by assisting her with the drawing so that she is successful. Mix easy tasks (making a dot on the page) with more difficult ones (drawing a vertical line) to maintain motivation.	Continue to increase the difficulty of the task (moving to circle, plus sign and square), using the same strategies.
During small-group time, Saul will attend to the teacher while she reads a story for the duration of the story.	Begin by having Saul choose the story or help a friend choose the story. Start with very short periods of time. Reward Saul by having him play an active role (e.g., getting to turn the page) or giving him a cut-out picture from the story that he can hold for each minute he is attending. Find an aspect of the story he likes and have him act it out. Other children can take turns doing these things as well, to provide appropriate models.	Increase the amount of time Saul needs to pay attention before getting his direct reward. Once he is doing well, he can be required to attend to something of another student's choosing before he gets to choose a story.
Julia will count, recognize numerals, and find appropriate quantities for the numbers 1–20, and count objects with 1:1 correspondence up to 20.	An initial assessment indicates that Julia is beginning to recognize numerals and can count by rote to 10. To help her with 1:1 correspondence, you can begin by having her count objects she likes—for example, the number of pieces in a puzzle, the number of crackers she would like to eat at snack time, or the number of pictures on the page of her favorite book. Her counting can then be directly reinforced with access to the item she has counted. Similarly, she can learn to match written numerals to groups of favored items or pictures of something she likes.	Use the same strategies listed above with increased complexity to increase Julia's counting skills and quantity identification. She may enjoy being a helper and sorting papers or pencils into piles of 20 (the number of children in the classroom) for the teacher. She may get to choose the manipulative she will work with when matching numerals to quantities.

(cont.)

TABLE 5.8. *(cont.)*

Sample annual IEP goal or curriculum area	Where to begin	How to move forward
Peter will identify and categorize items based on whether they are plant, mammal, bird, or fish, with 80% accuracy.	It is likely that several students are working on understanding the differences between plants and animals, as well as among different types of animals. Working together in a group to play a game that categorizes pictures of play objects can be a fun way to teach this concept if Peter is motivated by interacting with other students. If Peter likes playing in water, he can categorize objects by placing them in a box, water table, can, or cup. For every five objects he categorizes correctly, he can then play with the objects and containers in the water. He may do this in a group of other students who enjoy water, and thus he can work on social goals during this time as well.	Once Peter can categorize easily in situations you set up, he can begin to practice this skill in other settings. If he wants to join a game of kickball on the playground, you can require him to tell you if the grass is a plant or animal before moving on. You can actively involve him in listening to a story or lesson by asking him to categorize story characters or creatures. Other students may have stickers or t-shirts with animals or birds on them that he can categorize before getting to play with the student.
Amir will name and give values to units of money with 80% accuracy, both at school and on community outings.	You may need to begin working on this goal as a matching task. Have Amir match coins and paper money that are alike. He can then trade the coins for items he wants to "buy." Give another student some of Amir's favorite items for him to "buy" with his matched coins.	As Amir learns to match, he can learn the value of each coin. He can then trade the coins for items he wants to "buy," which you have now labeled with a purchase price.
Mei Lein will use writing in a functional context with assistance, as measured by her ability to answer written questions with complete sentences, 80% of the time over 2 trial days.	Mei Lein may begin by learning to write her name and commonly used words. She can write her name on some paper and use that paper to label items she wants to play with. She can use other written words to request items she wants (e.g., *BALL, CAR, SWING, COOKIE*). These can be traded for the item she wants. She can copy sentences from an article or book that has information about a topic she enjoys, and she can then be rewarded by being allowed to talk about that topic.	Mei Lein can then learn to write full sentences to respond to questions or to request items she wants.
Caroline will learn to read a map to find North, South, East, West, and the states of the United States with 80% accuracy over 2 trial days.	Caroline can begin to learn directions when she is moving about the classroom and playground. For example, if she would like to leave her desk to go to the art area, she needs to look at a "map" of the classroom and let you know if she will be moving North, South, East, or West to get to her next destination.	To learn the states, Caroline may begin with a puzzle of the United States to help her identify where each state is. She may need to find out interesting information about each state and match that to the state on the map. For example, if she really enjoys a specific TV show, she can find the state in which it is set, and the home states for each of the characters. If she likes ice cream, she can identify which states consume or produce the most ice cream. This can be done with other students as a team, to increase motivation and teach cooperative learning.

CHAPTER 6
Integrating CPRT into Your Classroom

CHAPTER OVERVIEW

Now that you are familiar with the components of CPRT, you are ready to learn more about strategies that make CPRT work in the classroom. A primary challenge of using CPRT is integrating it with your current classroom elements, such as your curriculum, school standards, and other intervention approaches. CPRT does not contain its own curriculum because its components are designed to make it a teaching tool applicable to a wide range of content. Several other interventions for children with autism are compatible with CPRT, and this chapter provides ways to integrate these strategies optimally into your classroom. Several methods of data collection are described for use with CPRT, as it is crucial to assess progress toward goals and standards in order to plan ongoing instruction. Identifying motivating materials through preference assessments, and encouraging generalization of skills through constant variation, are reviewed. Finally, the chapter provides troubleshooting tips for integrating CPRT into your classroom.

The following sections are included:

Using CPRT with School-Based Standards
    Using CPRT with Other Curricula
    Using CPRT with Classroom Themes

Integrating CPRT with Other Intervention Strategies
    Maintaining Fidelity of Implementation
    Interventions Compatible with CPRT
    How to Integrate Multiple Interventions

Identifying Motivating Materials
    Gathering Information
    Conducting a Preference Assessment

Collecting Data during CPRT
    Getting Started
    Data Collection Sheets

Using CPRT to Encourage Generalization

Troubleshooting

This chapter has a corresponding training lecture on the DVD accompanying this manual (*CPRT Session 4: Tracking Student Progress*).

Using CPRT
with School-Based Standards

Your decisions about what curricula to use in your classroom may be based on a variety of factors. You may be able to choose a curriculum, or you may be required to teach certain standards to your students. Because lessons and standards typically vary from one school district to the next, CPRT does not contain a recommended curriculum.

CPRT components are designed to be universally applicable and relevant to your current classroom goals.

Using CPRT with Other Curricula

Because there is no specific curriculum for CPRT, it is better to think of CPRT as a method for teaching within the curriculum you are already using. Similar to the way activities can be adapted in CPRT to meet IEP goals, specific curriculum activities can be modified if CPRT is appropriate. CPRT may be especially helpful for students who are not making progress with the standard teaching methods. CPRT principles can be used to make activities more motivating and instructions clearer for students who need added support.

Using CPRT
with Classroom Themes

In addition to standardized curricula, many teachers use theme-based teaching as part of their classroom program. CPRT strategies can easily be incorporated into theme-based activities.

Using CPRT with themes requires thinking about aspects of a theme that are motivating for the class and particular stu-

dents. Using the principles of CPRT can also help determine how long a theme might last. For example, if the class is really interested in the "Community Helpers" theme because the students enjoy learning about different occupations, it might be a good idea to extend this theme and integrate it into teaching social interaction, object play, and academic skills. Alternatively, if a majority of the class is no longer interested in "Community Helpers," you may need to alter your approach to the theme. It may be better to shorten the amount of time spent on the theme or to integrate more motivating activities. For example, integrating the vehicles used by each occupation may spark the interest of students who like to play with cars but have become bored with the "Community Helper" theme.

 Two forms for identifying motivating materials are available in *Part IV—Handout 4: Time-Based Preference Assessment*, and *Handout 5: Paired-Choice Preference Assessment*. These are discussed later in this chapter.

Integrating CPRT with Other
Intervention Strategies

Most teachers report that they use several different strategies in their classrooms to best meet their students' needs. It is unrealistic and inappropriate to assume that a single approach can universally apply to all your students in all possible situations. Therefore, CPRT can be successfully incorporated into your current repertoire of teaching methodologies. However, this integration should be done with care and attention to the integrity of each individual methodology.

Maintaining Fidelity of Implementation

Fidelity of implementation is the degree to which an intervention is implemented in the ways it was intended to be. Measuring fidelity of implementation is important in both research studies and clinical use. CPRT has considerable research support, meaning that it has been tested repeatedly and has been shown to be successful in helping students learn. However, this success has been demonstrated when CPRT is implemented correctly and in its entirety. In other words, there has been good fidelity of implementation, or good treatment adherence. It is not clear how students will benefit from CPRT if only certain components are used or if the components are not used correctly. So when research supports an intervention like CPRT, it essentially means that certain components, when used together and when used correctly, will be beneficial for teaching students. For this reason, it is important to fully understand each intervention you use before attempting to integrate it in your teaching.

Interventions Compatible with CPRT

CPRT is a naturalistic behavioral intervention, which means that it is based on the principles of ABA and has been developed for use in the natural environment. Many other popular, research-supported interventions share this behavioral base. For example, Discrete Trial Teaching (DTT) is a well-known behavioral intervention for educating children with autism. DTT is typically more structured and does not share essential design components with CPRT; CPRT is designed to be used in natural learning environments and to deliver reinforcement in a natural way. Interventions such as the Picture Exchange Communication System (PECS), and Milieu and Incidental Teaching, are much more similar to CPRT in this respect. *Figure 6.1* highlights several naturalistic behavioral interventions. If you are already comfortable using these or similar approaches, you may find that it is easy to incorporate CPRT into your teaching. Developmental or relationship-based strategies such as the Denver Model and DIR/ Floortime share some strategies with CPRT as well, such as following the student's lead, taking turns, responding to purposeful communication (rewarding attempts), and

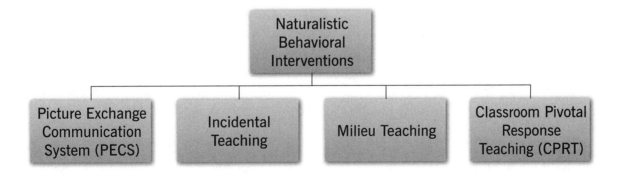

FIGURE 6.1. Examples of Naturalistic Behavioral Interventions. All of these approaches share some strategies and can be implemented during day-to-day classroom activities.

using natural reinforcement. These behavioral and developmental interventions may vary in their level of structure and the specific steps, but there are also many similarities among these approaches.

 See *Chapter 2* for a complete description of the principles of ABA.

You may use other specific strategies that are not part of a manualized intervention program. For example, some students benefit from additional environmental support, such as the use of a picture schedule to organize their day or a song to signal transitions. Although these strategies are not part of CPRT, they do not interfere with CPRT either. A student can use a choice board to choose the toy she wishes to play with, and then CPRT strategies can be used to expand on play with that toy. A teacher may use DTT to teach a student to identify pictures of all the students in his class, and CPRT during snack time to have him gain his peers' attention by using their names.

One important consideration is how you will clearly define for yourself and other classroom staff members which strategies should be used and when. Because various interventions only share some components, there are a few elements that are not compatible. This may lead to confusion for your students. For example, PECS and CPRT are very similar in concept, but PECS teaches communication through pictures, and CPRT typically teaches verbal or signed communication. If you use both these strategies in your classroom, it must be clear to your students when each type of communication is expected, or else clear that you will accept either form at any time. Another example involves DTT and CPRT. Although these two interventions share a common behavioral base, DTT relies primarily on indirect reinforcement, and CPRT employs

direct reinforcement. If you are alternating between these two interventions, you must have appropriate materials to reinforce your students' behavior. There may be times when one intervention is more effective than others for particular students or for teaching specific skills.

 See the *Component 6: Direct Reinforcement* section of *Chapter 3* for a complete description of providing reinforcement related to an activity.

How to Integrate Multiple Interventions

There are three recommended ways to integrate multiple interventions into your teaching. These options are described below.

Use Different Strategies for Different Activities

Some teachers find that it works best to use specific interventions to teach during certain activities. For example, you may use PECS during an art activity, and CPRT during circle time, one-on-one teaching, and facilitated play time. Alternatively, you may find that DTT works best when you are teaching self-help skills or new concepts that require memorized rote responses, such as multiplication tables. Similarly, you may find that it is most effective to use different teaching strategies for different parts of a teaching activity. You may use indirect reinforcement strategies such as tokens (which are not part of CPRT) when you reward students for paying attention while you explain a new math concept. Then, during their independent math time, you may use CPRT by providing a choice of materials, taking turns completing problems, and interspersing easy and difficult skills.

Use Different Strategies for Different Students

Another method for integrating interventions involves using different strategies for different students within activities. For example, you might find that many of your students learn best through CPRT, but that some students respond more readily to DTT. When structuring activities, you may interact with these students by using these different procedures. For example, during time on the playground, you may teach John using DTT and Noah using CPRT. If you are teaching the students to jump off a low platform, you may reinforce John's attempt to jump (even though it wasn't perfect) by allowing him to choose another activity on the play structure (direct reinforcement). When Noah steps off the platform instead of jumping, you tell him to "try again" and help him to climb back up. After several tries, Noah jumps, so you give him a high five and a sticker of his favorite character. Although the activity is the same, you have decided ahead of time that these two students will be taught using different interventions. If you find that CPRT does not work well with a student to teach a particular skill, it doesn't mean that CPRT doesn't work for that student overall. It may still be the most effective strategy for teaching a different skill. As you become familiar with new students, you will be able to determine more readily when a particular intervention will or will not work well.

Use Different Strategies for Different Goals or Types of Goals

A final strategy for integrating interventions involves using different teaching strategies to target different types of goals. Some learning goals may naturally lend themselves to being taught via CPRT, while others may be difficult to teach using these components. For example, CPRT calls for using direct reinforcement strategies and turn taking. These strategies may be difficult to incorporate into teaching self-help skills such as potty training. If a student does not find anything fun or motivating associated with potty training, then you will need to rely on indirect reinforcement.

Figure 6.2 highlights the optimal ways of utilizing multiple interventions with the students in your classroom.

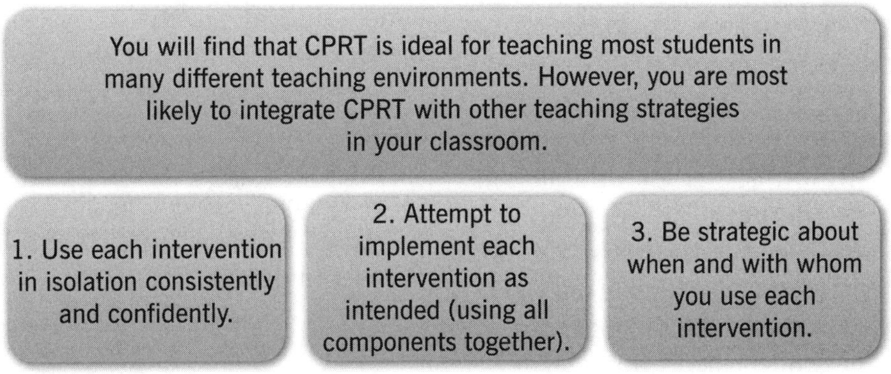

You will find that CPRT is ideal for teaching most students in many different teaching environments. However, you are most likely to integrate CPRT with other teaching strategies in your classroom.

1. Use each intervention in isolation consistently and confidently.

2. Attempt to implement each intervention as intended (using all components together).

3. Be strategic about when and with whom you use each intervention.

FIGURE 6.2. Integrating Interventions. This figure highlights the important points regarding integrating multiple interventions in your classroom.

Identifying Motivating Materials

Maximizing your students' motivation is an essential part of using CPRT. For this reason, it is important that you assess which activities, materials, sounds, textures, or snacks are preferred by each of your students. There are many ways you can figure out what a student likes when you first welcome her into your classroom. Because your students' likes and dislikes will probably change over time, reassess their preferences on a regular basis throughout the school year.

Gathering Information

Parents, former teachers, and other service providers will have valuable information on what techniques and tools they have used to motivate your students. You will want to find out about materials each student enjoys, as well as activities or topics of conversation that are motivating. It is also important to know about any stereotyped or self-stimulatory behaviors that may be used as reinforcers.

Find out about materials the student enjoys, as well as activities or topics of conversation that are motivating.

Take note of not only which materials work well as rewards, but also the details of how the reinforcement is delivered. Sometimes the specific materials are not as important as *how* an adult uses them. For example, your student's father may report that the student loves toy airplanes. However, after observing the pair playing together, you realize that the student loves how her father zooms the airplanes into her tummy for tickles and how he crashes the

airplanes together. Another consideration is how your student enjoys playing with a toy on her own. You may think that putting puzzle pieces into the frame should be the most enjoyable part of the activity, but your student may enjoy removing each piece or dumping all the pieces onto the table. Additionally, your student may have very specific interests regarding certain materials or snacks. She may love red candies but dislike green ones, or she may enjoy lying across a therapy ball but dislike bouncing on it. As you gather information, be aware of what specifically motivates your students. Ask for detailed information from your coworkers and your students' parents. You may want to distribute copies of *Handout 3: Gathering Information* to other adults who know your students well. See *Figure 6.3* for a completed example of this form; a reproducible blank copy of the handout is provided in *Part IV*.

Conducting a Preference Assessment

As noted in *Chapters 1 and 2*, a preference assessment is a formal and systematic way of gathering information on what your student enjoys. There are various methods for conducting a preference assessment. Two options are outlined here: time-based preference assessment and paired-choice preference assessment. You may find that you prefer to use the time-based type to determine preferred toys and activities, and the paired-choice type to determine preferred foods and drinks.

Preference assessments are an effective way to determine individual likes and dislikes.

| HANDOUT 3 | **Gathering Information** | |

Student: **Saul**

We need your help! We know that your experience with **Saul**
will be very helpful as we welcome him/her into our classroom. Please take a few minutes to tell us what he/
she likes. Be specific. We will use this information to keep him/her motivated to learn and interested in classroom
activities. Thank you for your help!

Completed by: **Ms. Jones**   Relationship to student: **Previous teacher**

What does he/she enjoy?

What	How	How much (3 = high)	When
Example: Playing on computer (alphabet game)	*Likes to match capital to lower-case letters (alone only; has trouble sharing)*	1 ② 3	*Good as a transition back to classroom after lunch or morning recess*
Example: Graham crackers	*Whole or half crackers; rejects crackers that are broken unevenly*	1 2 ③	*Any time*
Spaghetti ball (sensory ball)	Stretching the strings while naming the colors	1 2 ③	Morning transition into the classroom; favorite first activity
Water play	Enjoys splashing water with palms and putting forearms under water	1 ② 3	Any time; will be motivated for water incorporated into any activity
Blue's Clues	Likes to sing along to the songs on the *Blue's Clues* radio toy	1 2 ③	Works well as a break between two more structured, academic-type tasks
Gummi bears	Likes all colors	1 2 ③	Useful for extremely nonpreferred tasks, such as toothbrushing and potty
Elephants	Stickers and making elephant noises	1 ② 3	Any time; watching someone else pretend to be an elephant is also motivating
Matchbox cars	Primarily spins wheels or opens/closes doors if possible	① 2 3	Free-play time; will roll cars with a model, but spins wheels if left alone
		1 2 3	

Any other tips or comments? **Saul often takes several seconds to make a decision when offered choices. Providing him**
extra time to choose can help.

FIGURE 6.3. Completed Example of *Handout 3: Gathering Information*. On this form, Saul's old teacher has listed several toys and activities that Saul enjoyed during his time in her class. She has also provided helpful tips about working with Saul in her comments.

Time-Based Preference Assessment

A time-based preference assessment allows you to observe how your student interacts with different materials when given a free opportunity to do so. Based on observations and information from others, select 10 items you believe the student will enjoy. For example, you may select the top items or activities on the copies of *Handout 3: Gathering Information* that you have asked the student's parents and former teachers to fill out. Also, take into account what materials or activities have been popular with other students in your class. Consider items with varied features (e.g., textures, sounds, functions).

Set aside 5 minutes to conduct the assessment with your student. Choose an area in your room that is free from distraction and other items. The goal is to determine how the student will respond to the specific materials you have selected, so nothing else should interfere. During the assessment, record what your student is doing at predetermined intervals. For example, you may set a timer to sound every 10 seconds. When the timer goes off, record which items the student is using and how he is using it. You may find that the student plays with one or two toys for the entire 5 minutes! If this occurs, rest assured that you have accurately identified something he likes. However, you may want to conduct an additional assessment with these highly preferred items excluded, in order to determine what other materials may also be preferred to a lesser extent. Record your findings on *Handout 4: CPRT Time-Based Preference Assessment*. A completed example of this form is shown in *Figure 6.4*; a reproducible blank copy is provided in *Part IV.*

Paired-Choice Preference Assessment

A paired-choice assessment allows you to observe how your student interacts with different materials when presented with a series of choices. Based on observation and information from others, select six items you believe the student will enjoy. As mentioned above, you may select the top items or activities on the copies of *Handout 3: Gathering Information* you have collected. Also, again, take into account what items have been popular with other students in your class, and consider items with varied features (e.g., textures, tastes, colors).

During the assessment, set up a series of trials in which pairs of items are set in front of the student. Allow the student to make a choice between the two items (e.g., reaching, gaze shift, verbal request), and remove the other item. Record the choice while the student consumes the food item or plays with the toy. If the student does not make a choice, remove both items and re-present them in a later trial. If the student attempts to take both items, block the attempt and re-present the pair in a later trial. Record your findings on *Handout 5: CPRT Paired-Choice Preference Assessment*. A completed example of this form is shown in *Figure 6.5*; a reproducible blank copy is provided in *Part IV.*

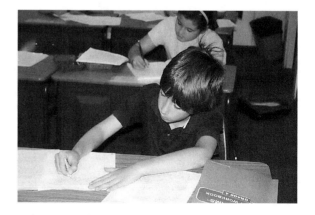

| HANDOUT 4 | **CPRT Time-Based Preference Assessment** | |

Student: _Saul_ _____ Date: _10/11/09_ _____

Choose a set of 10 items available in your classroom that you think the student might like. List each item (toy, food item, etc.) below.

Items	Number of times chosen	Rank
1. Spaghetti ball	9	2
2. Blue's Clues pop-up	2	6
3. Gummi bears	3*	1
4. Elephant figurine	2	7
5. Matchbox cars	3	4
6. Water wheel	3	5
7. Crayons and paper	0	10
8. Magnetic fish and pole	2	8
9. Inset circus animal puzzle	1	9
10. Light spinner	5	3

Ranked items	Preference level
Gummi bears	High
Spaghetti ball	High
Light spinner	High
Matchbox cars	Medium
Water wheel	Medium
Blue's Clues pop-up	Medium
Elephant figurine	Low
Fish and pole	Low
Circus puzzle	Low
Crayons	Low

Gather all the items, and make them all easily accessible to the student. Prior to the assessment, allow the student to try each of the items. Set a timer to sound every 10 seconds. When the timer goes off, indicate which item(s) the student is playing with or consuming by circling the number that corresponds with the item listed above. Replenish any food items during the assessment if necessary.

Interval	Item engaged with (circle)
1	1 2 ③ 4 5 6 7 8 9 10
2	1 2 ③ 4 5 6 7 8 9 10
3	1 2 ③ 4 5 6 7 8 9 10
4	① 2 3 4 5 6 7 8 9 10
5	① 2 3 4 5 6 7 8 9 10
6	① 2 3 4 5 6 7 8 9 10
7	① 2 3 4 5 6 7 8 9 10
8	1 2 3 4 5 6 7 ⑧ 9 10
9	1 2 3 4 5 6 7 ⑧ 9 10
10	1 2 3 4 5 6 7 8 ⑨ 10
11	1 2 3 4 5 ⑥ 7 8 9 10
12	1 ② 3 4 5 6 7 8 9 10
13	1 2 3 4 ⑤ 6 7 8 9 10
14	1 2 3 4 ⑤ 6 7 8 9 10
15	1 2 3 4 ⑤ 6 7 8 9 10

Interval	Item engaged with (circle)
16	① 2 3 4 5 6 7 8 9 10
17	① 2 3 4 5 6 7 8 9 10
18	① 2 3 4 5 6 7 8 9 10
19	1 2 3 ④ 5 6 7 8 9 10
20	1 2 3 ④ 5 6 7 8 9 10
21	1 2 3 4 5 6 7 8 9 ⑩
22	1 2 3 4 5 6 7 8 9 ⑩
23	1 2 3 4 5 6 7 8 9 ⑩
24	1 2 3 4 5 6 7 8 9 ⑩
25	1 2 3 4 5 6 7 8 9 ⑩
26	1 ② 3 4 5 6 7 8 9 10
27	1 2 3 4 5 ⑥ 7 8 9 10
28	1 2 3 4 5 ⑥ 7 8 9 10
29	① 2 3 4 5 6 7 8 9 10
30	① 2 3 4 5 6 7 8 9 10

Count the number of time points at which the student was engaged with each item. Then rank the items from the most often selected to the least often. Highly preferred items are the three items the student selected most often, moderately preferred items are the three items selected the next most often, and so forth (see scale on right).

Other notes: _*Did not replenish gummi bears after first 30 seconds to promote interest in other items gummi bears highly preferred._
Enjoyed exploring all available items; moved quickly among choices.
_____
_____

FIGURE 6.4. Completed Example of *Handout 4: CPRT Time-Based Preference Assessment*. Using this form, Saul's teacher has collected information on what toys and activities are particularly motivating to Saul. She used several items listed by Saul's previous teacher on *Handout 3: Gathering Information* (see *Figure 6.3*), as well as presenting several new items. All the items were available to Saul throughout the assessment, and he was allowed to play freely with the items of his choice. Notice that the teacher ranked gummi bears as the most preferred (Rank 1) because she noticed that Saul preferred these exclusively at the beginning of the assessment. She wrote a comment in the "Other notes" section to explain that she stopped offering the gummi bears after the first 30 seconds to promote interest in other toys.

| HANDOUT 5 | **CPRT Paired-Choice Preference Assessment** | |

Student: **Saul** _____   Date: **10/11/09** _____

Choose a set of six items available in your classroom that you think the student might like. List each item (toy, food item, etc.) below. Gather all items so they are easily accessible throughout the assessment.

Stimulus	Percent chosen	Preference level		
1. Spaghetti ball	**8** /10 = **80** %	(High)	Medium	Low
2. *Blue's Clues* pop-up	**1** /10 = **10** %	High	Medium	(Low)
3. Gummi bears	**9** /10 = **90** %	(High)	Medium	Low
4. Elephant figurine	**4** /10 = **40** %	High	(Medium)	Low
5. Matchbox cars	**4** /10 = **40** %	High	(Medium)	Low
6. Water wheel	**4** /10 = **40** %	High	(Medium)	Low

On each trial, select the two items associated with the item numbers listed below. Place both items in front of the student. Record each item the student selects from the pair, and allow the student to interact briefly with the item. If the student does not select either item, pause the assessment and present each item one at a time, prompting the student to interact with it if necessary. Then re-present the trial. If the student does not select either item on the second presentation of the pair, move on. Block any attempts to access both items by removing the items and re-presenting the pair later in the assessment.

Trial	Left	Right	Item selected
1	1	2	Spaghetti ball
2	3	4	Gummi bears
3	5	6	Water wheel
4	2	3	Gummi bears
5	4	5	Elephant figurine
6	1	3	Gummi bears
7	2	4	Elephant figurine
8	3	5	Gummi bears
9	4	6	Water wheel
10	1	4	Spaghetti ball
11	3	6	Water wheel
12	2	5	Matchbox cars
13	6	1	Spaghetti ball
14	1	5	Spaghetti ball
15	2	6	Water wheel

Trial	Left	Right	Item selected
16	4	1	Spaghetti ball
17	6	3	Gummi bears
18	5	2	Matchbox cars
19	1	6	Spaghetti ball
20	5	1	Spaghetti ball
21	6	2	*Blue's Clues* pop-up
22	2	1	Spaghetti ball
23	4	3	Gummi bears
24	6	5	Matchbox cars
25	3	2	Gummi bears
26	5	4	Matchbox cars
27	3	1	Gummi bears
28	4	2	Elephant figurine
29	5	3	Gummi bears
30	6	4	Elephant figurine

Calculate the percent of trials in which the student selected each item. Each item was presented 10 times. The percentage of trials in which an item was selected can be determined by dividing the number of times the item was selected by 10. Highly preferred items are those selected in 80% or more of the trials. Moderately preferred items are those selected in 40–70%. Low-preference items are selected in less than 40% of the trials.

Other notes: **Tried to access water inside water wheel and lost interest when unable.** _____

_____

_____

FIGURE 6.5. Completed Example of *Handout 5: CPRT Paired-Choice Preference Assessment.* This form illustrates another example of how Saul's teacher may assess his preferences when he enters a new classroom. Here the teacher has taken the items listed on the *Gathering Information* worksheet by Saul's old teacher and presented them in matched pairs. She has then recorded Saul's choice from each pair and presented the next set.

Reassessment as Necessary

Student preferences will change throughout the school year. Plan to reassess preferences on a regular basis (monthly or bimonthly), or more frequently if you have difficulty motivating your student. Also, if you notice that attention or motivation is waning for a particular student, reassess her preferences to be sure you are maximizing her motivation.

Collecting Data during CPRT

Recording and analyzing information about your students' behavior are essential for maximizing learning and tracking progress. Teachers are often required to take data to ensure that the strategies being used are working, and that students are meeting IEP and curriculum goals. However, the process of collecting data is too often confusing, time-consuming, and awkward. Moreover, many of the data collected in clinics and classrooms are never reviewed to inform instruction or to determine what students are learning. This can be frustrating! In this part of the chapter, we make a few recommendations about data collection and tracking methods that have worked well for teachers using CPRT. In order to capture student progress regularly and to help modify goals as needed, we recommend collecting data on each goal at least once per week.

Getting Started

Before and throughout the process of gathering data, consider the following questions:

1. What information are you trying to capture?
2. What measurement criteria are written into each student's IEP goals?

3. What does your district or supervisor require?
4. What is manageable for you and other classroom staff members?
5. What information do you need to determine how to alter the student's program for maximal progress?

Data Collection Sheets

After you have developed a clear picture of what data are needed, you are ready to select specific data collection methods. Forms intended for quarterly planning, weekly or monthly analysis, and daily data collection are provided in *Part IV*. These forms should be used together to create a streamlined system for data collection/analysis and long-term planning. The forms, and the ways in which they work together, are discussed in the following sections.

CPRT Planning and Progress

Handout 6: CPRT Planning and Progress allows you to record all IEP goals and curriculum areas you plan to target by using CPRT with an individual student. This is the first form to be filled out when you decide to use CPRT with a student, as it allows you to identify which of the student's goals you will target with CPRT and think about activities that may be ideally suited for each goal. First, list the student's goals in the left-hand column. In the next column, list activities and settings that may be appropriate for working on each goal. This is not intended to limit the number of places the goal can be addressed, but instead to remind you to pay particular attention to the goal during these activities and possibly take data as well. For each goal, you then enter the date the goal was introduced. As the student spends time in your class, you will return to this form to update progress by noting which goals have been achieved, which are ongoing, and which (if any) have been discontinued.

The time points at which you transfer information to the *CPRT Planning and Progress* form are called Progress Assessments. The information to enter on this form is taken from *Handout 7: CPRT Goal Summary*, which provides details on each of the student's individual goals. (This handout is discussed in the next section.) There is room for three Progress Assessments on the *CPRT Planning and Progress* form. After three Progress Assessments, it will be necessary to transfer any unmet goals to a new copy of this form. If several goals have been achieved, new goals can be added. We recommend referencing this form approximately quarterly (once every 10–12 weeks) or at any time a goal has been met. A completed example of *Handout: CPRT Planning and Progress* is shown in *Figure 6.6*, with information for a student named Julia. Several of the completed-example forms in this chapter track Julia's progress on her goals, in order to show how the forms may be used together.

CPRT Goal Summary

Handout 7: CPRT Goal Summary allows you to specify details on each of the student's goals that will be targeted with CPRT. Here you can outline specific steps, or benchmarks, toward each primary goal. Each benchmark should contribute toward the accomplishment of the goal and should be measurable. On this form, you first enter the overall goal at the top of the form. Then each specific benchmark, or prompt level, is entered in the left-hand column of the form. Next to each benchmark, individual data points (taken from the *CPRT Data Record* forms, discussed below) are entered. These allow you to evaluate student progress on the benchmark or step after 4 days of data

collection. Four data collection days may span 1–2 weeks, depending on how often you collect data in your classroom.

The amount of time it takes to collect data four times is called a Period. The number of Periods a student needs to reach a particular benchmark or step will depend on the difficulty of the goal. This form makes it easy to see if a student is making progress over time, if a student is ready to move to the next benchmark, or if something needs to be changed to help the student meet a difficult goal. A completed example of *Handout 7: CPRT Goal Summary* is shown in *Figure 6.7*, with information on Julia's goal to label 5–10 new items per month. Again, the information to enter on this form is taken from the *CPRT Data Record* forms, which provide details on the student's day-to-day performance of the benchmark skills. These forms are discussed next.

CPRT Data Records

The *CPRT Data Record* forms allow you to take detailed data on individual student progress during or immediately after a CPRT interaction. There are several of these forms, and each provides a different level of detail on student performance. This allows you to collect data consistently, but to do so in a way that fits the context of a given interaction. It is important to think about the function each form can serve in your classroom as you utilize the different ways to collect student data. You may want to use different forms for different goals or activities. Alternatively, you may find that one form fits your classroom well, and you may use that form exclusively.

CPRT DATA RECORD: UNSTRUCTURED

Handout 8: CPRT DATA Record: Unstructured allows you to record when CPRT is used with a student to target specific goals.

HANDOUT 6		**CPRT Planning and Progress**

Student: **Julia**

This form is designed to facilitate planning and progress tracking related to IEP goals and curriculum areas. Enter goals that can be optimally targeted using CPRT on the grid below. For each goal, think of 1–3 classroom settings or activities in which this goal can be addressed with CPRT. List the activity ideas and the date of goal introduction in the spaces provided. **Each month**, mark the date of the Progress Assessment (PA) and review the relevant *CPRT Goal Summary* sheets for the specified goals. If the student has met the goal, circle A for Achieved and draw a line through the remaining PA columns. If the student is making progress but has not yet met the mastery criteria for a particular goal, circle O for Ongoing and continue addressing the goal through CPRT. If a student is not making progress on a goal despite correct and consistent implementation of CPRT, circle D for Discontinue and consider alternative strategies to reach this goal. Transfer Ongoing goals to a new *CPRT Planning and Progress* sheet after three Progress Assessments.

KEY

A: Achieved; student has met mastery criteria for this goal.

O: Ongoing; student is making progress, and the goal will continue to be addressed through CPRT.

D: Discontinue; student is making no progress on this goal; consider alternative strategies.

IEP or Curriculum Area Goal	Activities/Settings	Date Introduced	PA 1 Date: 12/15	PA 2 Date: 3/05	PA 3 Date:
Use 5–10 new labels to request per month; use in 2 settings w/2 people	Snack, art, play, outside time	9/12/08	A Ⓞ D	Ⓐ O D	A O D
Learn 5 new representational play actions, 3-step sequences	Play, circle time	9/12/08	A Ⓞ D	A Ⓞ D	A O D
Participate in familiar play theme with peer	Play, small groups, reading	9/12/08	A Ⓞ D	A Ⓞ D	A O D
Count, recognize numerals, find quantities for 1–20	Circle time, snack, gross motor	9/12/08	Ⓐ O D	A O D	A O D
			A O D	A O D	A O D
			A O D	A O D	A O D
			A O D	A O D	A O D

FIGURE 6.6. Completed Example of *Handout 6: CPRT Planning and Progress*. On this form, Julia's teacher has planned which of Julia's goals she will target with CPRT. The teacher has chosen labeling, learning new play actions, themed play with a peer, and counting. For each of these goals, she has entered several activities that lend themselves to targeting these goals with Julia, and the date she introduced each goal. The teacher has completed two Progress Assessments with information taken from *Handout 7: CPRT Goal Summary* for each individual goal. This form clearly summarizes Julia's progress on her goals and can be used to share progress with parents, administrators, and the IEP team.

HANDOUT 7

CPRT Goal Summary

Student: **Julia**

This form is designed to track student progress on goals being addressed with CPRT. Write the curriculum area or IEP goal in the space provided, and enter the first step to reaching the goal in the grid below. Enter the date that this benchmark or step was introduced. On each data collection day, transfer data from one of the *CPRT Data Records* to this sheet. Depending on which *CPRT Data Record* was used, enter the plus/check/minus rating and support level typically required to elicit the target skill (from *CPRT Data Record: Unstructured* or *CPRT Data Record: Semistructured*) or the exact measurement of goal progress (from *CPRT Data Record: Structured*). After four data collection days (a Period), use the measurements listed to determine if the step is Achieved (A) or Ongoing (O), and circle the appropriate option. This will allow you to assess progress on the goal over time and to determine necessary next steps for your student and teaching staff.

Goal: **Julia will use 5–10 new labels per month to make requests.**

Benchmark/Step or Procedure Changes		Period 1				A O	Period 2				A O	Period 3				A O	Period 4				A O
		1	2	3	4		1	2	3	4		1	2	3	4		1	2	3	4	
Hold motivating item up. Provide verbal models (FV)	Date	10/9	10/10	10/12	10/13	A Ⓞ	10/16	10/19	10/20	10/23	A Ⓞ	10/24	10/25	10/27	10/28	A Ⓞ	10/29	10/30	10/31	11/1	Ⓐ O
	10/9	1/4	2/6	+/FV	1/4		1/6	–/FV	+/PV	2/5		+/FV	+/PV	3/4	4/6		6/7	4/4	5/6	3/3	
Hold item up. Provide initial sound (PV)	Date	11/4	11/5	11/6		A O					A O					A O					A O
	11/2	6/11	–/PV	1/6																	
Item in sight, out of reach. Point, provide initial sound (GP + PV)	Date					A O					A O					A O					A O
Item in sight but out of reach. Point and wait expectantly (GP)	Date					A O					A O					A O					A O
Item available	Date					A O					A O					A O					A O

FIGURE 6.7. Completed Example of *Handout 7: CPRT Goal Summary.* On this form, Julia's teacher has specified the benchmarks necessary for Julia to achieve her goal of using 5–10 new labels per month to make requests. As seen in this example, Julia's teacher first introduced the benchmark of repeating the label after a full verbal model on 10/9, and she has logged four Periods of data on this skill. During the first Period, Julia was labeling items correctly only on 25–33% of trials or opportunities, as demonstrated by the 1/4, 2/6, and 1/4 data points transferred to this form. The teacher has transferred these scores from *Handout 10: CPRT Data Record: Structured,* which tracks student response to each opportunity presented. The entry +/FV refers to mostly correct responding with a full verbal prompt, which is the least supportive prompt Julia needed to label items during the CPRT interaction on which the teacher took data. The teacher has transferred this data from *Handout 8: CPRT Data Record: Unstructured* or *Handout 9: CPRT Data Record: Semistructured,* either of which collects more general information about a student's behavior during a CPRT interaction. After the fourth Period, the benchmark of imitating a full verbal model to label an item was considered achieved, due to Julia's consistent performance of the skill at this level (she performed the skills 86–100% correctly during this period). The teacher has now moved on to collecting daily data on Julia's ability to use the label when she is only provided a partial verbal model (initial sound). She has collected data for nearly a full Period on this benchmark. If Julia had not achieved the initial benchmark within four Periods but was making consistent progress, the teacher might have continued data collection on this first benchmark by repeating the benchmark on the second row (all benchmarks are entered here for the purposes of illustration, but typically they would be entered as needed). If Julia was not making progress on this goal over the four Periods, the teacher would probably have considered an alternative strategy to CPRT to teach this skill.

The date of each interaction and the initials of the teacher or paraprofessional involved in the interaction are listed in the two left-hand columns. The activity, materials, and length of time of the interaction are listed next. Next, main goals for each interaction are entered on this data sheet, along with the student's acquisition and maintenance skills for the goals targeted. This information will allow you to examine possible reasons for progress or lack of progress. For example, perhaps the materials were not motivating, not enough time was spent on a specific goal, or the acquisition skills for the goal were too difficult. Entering this information before the interaction with your student will also give you a clear understanding of the best ways to present opportunities to respond to your student. After the interaction, you can use the form to record the level of the student's response to maintenance and acquisition skills, using a simple three-point system: a plus if the student is responding correctly most of the time, a check if the student is responding correctly some of the time, or a minus if the student is rarely or never responding correctly. In addition, you can list the types of prompts used to help your student respond. It may be helpful to jot down quick notes throughout the interaction in order to record the most accurate information.

The *CPRT Data Record: Unstructured* form may be useful for tracking progress on a daily basis to maintain consistency across your teaching staff. It allows each person working with the student to utilize the same maintenance and acquisition skills for similar goals. A completed example of this form is shown in *Figure 6.8.* To transfer the information on the *CPRT Data Record: Unstructured* form to the *CPRT Goal Summary* form, record the plus, check, or minus as well as the level of prompt needed for the student to respond correctly in the row

for the current benchmark. In general, the prompt level recorded here should match the level of the benchmark that the student is working on. If the level of prompt needed to use the skill is significantly more supportive than the current benchmark, this may be an indication to back up and focus more carefully on the student's ability to generalize and maintain the skill at that level. If the prompt needed to use the skill is significantly less supportive than the current benchmark, and the student is consistently performing the skill in many contexts, it may be time to move forward to the next, more difficult benchmark.

CPRT DATA RECORD: SEMISTRUCTURED

Handout 9: CPRT Data Record: Semistructured provides a simple way to record one student's response on benchmarks from several goals, and it is designed to follow your student throughout the day or across one day. The form is called "semistructured" because after working with your student for a few minutes, you pause and make notes on the form, and then continue with your teaching. You maintain this pattern throughout the teaching interaction. To use this form, select several benchmarks from various goals to target, and identify maintenance and acquisition skills for each one. Enter this information on the form in the spaces provided. Throughout the day, time spent targeting each of these benchmarks in several activities can be recorded on this form. Each time you address a particular goal, record the interaction in the table under the appropriate benchmark. Depending on how long the interaction lasts, you may record data only once during each activity (activities/interactions that last 5 minutes or less), or several times by pausing briefly throughout (every 3–5 minutes). At each data collection point, space is provided

CPRT Data Record: Unstructured

Student: _Julia_

To use this data record, complete one row each time you use CPRT with your student. This method does not require data collection during the interaction with the student. Complete the row at the end of the interaction, and note the length of the interaction in the appropriate column. Use the key below to indicate the student's general level of responding for both acquisition and maintenance skills, prompts used, and level of motivation and compliance.

KEY:

+ = Responds independently to all or almost all (at least 80%) opportunities

✓ = Responds independently to most opportunities (50%), but requires support for some opportunities

– = Requires support to respond to all or almost all opportunities

Prompt Level:
F: Full or **P:** Partial

Prompt Type:
Ph: Physical, **V:** Verbal, **Vs:** Visual, **G:** Gestural

Motivation/Compliance:
1—Optimal motivation, minimal negative behaviors
2—High motivation, few negative behaviors
3—Good motivation, some negative behaviors
4—Poor motivation, moderate negative behaviors
5—Minimal motivation, many negative behaviors

Date	Teacher	Activity/materials + length of time	Goal/curriculum area	Acquisition skills	+ ✓ –	Sample best acquisition skill response (include prompt level, if any)	Most frequent prompt level (if any)	Maintenance skills	+ ✓ –	Motivation
10/19	LR	Free play/train set, ~10 minutes	Representational play actions	Person on the train, washing the train	✓	Person on the train, waved good-bye (GP)	FG (model play actions)	Pushing the train down the track	+	1 2 ③ 4 5
10/19	HC	Snack time, pretzels and raisins, ~15 minutes	Single-word labels, novel items	Single words	–	"et-zel", initial sound as prompt (PV)	FV	Initial sounds to request	+	1 ② 3 4 5
10/19	LR	Outside play, play structure, ~10 minutes	Pretend with peer	Participating w/peer	✓	Followed peer's instructions	FG (point to peer)	Playing near peer, watches	+	1 2 3 ④ 5
10/20	JS	Art time, eyedropper painting, ~15 minutes	Single-word labels, colors	Identifying purple, orange, and green	+	"Green" independent, purple + orange with initial sound	PV	Red, yellow, blue	+	1 2 3 4 ⑤
10/21	JS	Free play, dolls, ~10 minutes	Pretend with peer	Feeding doll, sharing w/peer	+	Fed doll with bottle while peer held doll	None	Known actions, independent play with doll	+	1 2 3 4 ⑤

FIGURE 6.8. Completed Example of *Handout 8: CPRT Data Record: Unstructured.* On this form, Julia's teachers and the paraprofessionals in her classroom have recorded data during several CPRT interactions across 3 days. In these interactions, various goals are targeted in several activities, and you can see that Julia is consistently performing her maintenance skills in each area (score of "+"). Her use of acquisition skills is varied across activities, however. She is able to consistently use single words (score of "+") with a partial verbal (PV) model during art time, which is highly motivating for her (Motivation rating 5), but is less consistent and requires a full verbal model to use her labels during snack, which is less motivating (Motivation rating 2). It may be helpful to look at this form in conjunction with *Handout 7: CPRT Goal Summary* to understand how the data may be transferred. To transfer the data points regarding Julia's ability to label to the *CPRT Goal Summary* form, the teacher would enter "–/FV" for the date of the snack activity and "+/PV" for the date of the art activity (see 10/19 and 10/20 entries in Period 2 on *Handout 7: CPRT Goal Summary*). Though the "+/PV" entry indicates that Julia performed the skill correctly most of the time with a less supportive prompt than that specified by the current benchmark, the "–/FV" entry tells the teacher that she is not yet using this skill consistently in all contexts, and thus may need continued instruction at the current level of support.

to rate the student's responses to the acquisition tasks on the plus/check/minus scale, record the prompt level and type (by circling the appropriate letter), and list sample student acquisition responses. Also, maintenance task performance is rated on the plus/check/minus scale, to ensure consistent performance of these tasks and inform you of any adjustments that may need to be made (e.g., if the student is receiving a minus rating for maintenance skills on a particular benchmark across several activities, it may mean that you have moved forward with the goal too quickly). It is likely that the same activity may be entered under multiple target skills, because several of the student's goals may be addressed during a single activity.

This form is flexible and designed to collect data at a level of detail between the more anecdotal notes in *Handout 8: CPRT Data Record: Unstructured* and the detailed data from *Handout 10: CPRT Data Record: Structured* (see below). A completed example of the *CPRT Data Record: Semistructured* form is shown in *Figure 6.9*. Progress over time can be examined when data from several days are moved to *Handout 7: CPRT Goal Summary*. To transfer the information from to the *CPRT Goal Summary* form, record the plus/check/minus and the least supportive prompt from the end of each target skill grid. This represents the student's most frequent response level and the type of prompts the student needed to respond appropriately to the acquisition cue. Enter this information in the row of the current benchmark on the *CPRT Goal Summary* form. It is important to note that the Summary score should reflect the most consistent level of student response (e.g., if the student received a "+/FV" for two segments of the interaction but a "−/FV" for another, transfer the "+/FV" to the *CPRT Goal Summary* form, since this was more frequent). If there is an equal number of multiple response levels, transfer the student's best response.

CPRT DATA RECORD: STRUCTURED

Handout 10: CPRT Data Record: Structured allows you to document your student's responses in greater detail, as you record your student's behavior to each opportunity to respond for a particular goal. To use this form, first identify the goal and benchmark you are targeting with the student, and enter the maintenance and acquisition skills in the space provided. During the interaction, for each cue you provide to the student (called a trial), you circle whether the skill is a maintenance or acquisition skill for the student, and then circle how the student responds. There is also space to enter any support that is necessary to help the student respond successfully. A new column is used for each new cue (or trial) that you present to the student. Any important notes or comment regarding the interaction or the student's progress on the goal can be recorded at the bottom of each table within the form.

This method may be useful for tracking progress toward goals that specify a number or percentage of correct responses (e.g., 4 of 5 responses correct over 5 trial days, or 5 independent responses throughout the day). In order to track progress, only correct responses to acquisition goals at the appropriate level of support or better are counted as correct (e.g., if a student's benchmark for a particular goal specifies partial verbal support, then only correct trials with a partial verbal or less supportive model should be included in the student's score for the interaction). If appropriate to the goal, a percent correct can be calculated by dividing the number of correct acquisition responses into the total number of opportunities to use that skill. A score for the interaction is entered in the upper right-hand corner of the table. The type of score recorded will depend on the way the goal is written (e.g., if the goal requires 4 of 5 responses correct, then percent correct should be recorded

CPRT Data Record: Semistructured

Student: *Julia*   Date: *10/24*

To use this data record, record data during natural pauses in the activity every 3–5 minutes. **Before you begin CPRT:** Enter the goals to be addressed with CPRT in the spaces provided, and define maintenance and acquisition skills or targets for the student. **During the activity:** After each interval, record the materials and the type of support used *most often* to elicit the *acquisition skills*. Record sample student responses for the acquisition skills at the support level indicated. At each interval, rate the student's performance of maintenance skills for that goal, based on the key below.

Support Level:
F: Full or **P:** Partial

Support Type:
Ph: Physical, **V:** Verbal,
Vs: Visual, **G:** Gestural,
I: Independent (no support)

KEY:

+ = Responds independently to all or almost all (at least 80%) opportunities

✓ = Responds independently to most opportunities (50%), but requires support for some opportunities

– = Requires support to respond to all or almost all opportunities

Goal/Curriculum Area: *Use single-word labels for novel items to make requests.*

Maintenance Skill: Known words: *baby, phone, cookie*   **Acquisition Skill:** New words: *bottle, spoon, book, juice*

Initials	Material/Activity	Support		Acq. +/✓/–	Sample Student Response/Notes	Maint. +/✓/–
JS	Reading preferred books	ⓕ / P	Ph Ⓥ Vs G I	+	*Book, bird* (likes to flip pages)	+
JS	Reading preferred books	F / Ⓟ	Ph Ⓥ Vs G I	✓	*Book* (w/point) (made choice btw. 2)	+
HC	Structured play, babies	ⓕ / P	Ph Ⓥ Vs G I	✓	*Bottle, spoon* (likes to have materials)	+
HC	Structured play, babies	ⓕ / P	Ph Ⓥ Vs G I	+	*Spoon*	+
SUMMARY	Most frequent level of response:	+		Most frequent support level:	Full Verbal	

Goal/Curriculum Area: *Perform new representational play actions.*

Maintenance Skill: Known actions: *Carry doll, talk on toy phone (1 step)*   **Acquisition Skill:** *Feed doll (spoon and bottle), bathe baby, put baby to sleep*

Initials	Material/Activity	Support		Acq. +/✓/–	Sample Student Response/Notes	Maint. +/✓/–
LR	Structured play, babies	ⓕ / P	Ph V Vs Ⓖ I	–	Covered baby with blanket, "zzzzz" sound	+
LR	Structured play, babies/picnic	F / Ⓟ	Ph V Vs Ⓖ I	✓	Sat baby in front of plate, held food up	+
LR	Structured play, babies	F / Ⓟ	Ph V Vs Ⓖ I	✓	Covered with blanket, sang a song	+
		F / P	Ph V Vs G I			
SUMMARY	Most frequent level of response:	✓		Most frequent support level:	Partial Verbal	

(cont.)

FIGURE 6.9. Completed Example of *Handout 9: CPRT Data Record: Semistructured.* On this form, Julia's teachers and paraprofessionals in her classroom have recorded data during several CPRT interactions across one day. This form is more detailed than *Handout 8: CPRT Data Record: Unstructured*, but collects similar information. On some occasions, several goals are targeted in one activity (e.g., Julia's first three goals were all targeted during the structured play activity on 10/24). Also, during some activities the teacher or paraprofessional collected data multiple times (e.g., during reading preferred books activity and structured play with babies); for other activities, there was only one opportunity for recording (e.g., snack time). It may be helpful to look at this form in conjunction with *Handout 7: CPRT Goal Summary* to understand how the data may be transferred. The data on Julia's requesting skill from this example form have been transferred to Period 3 on the *CPRT Goal Summary* form. The teacher has

Goal/Curriculum Area: _Participate in rehearsed pretend theme play w/peer._

Maintenance Skill: _Parallel play near peer_   **Acquisition Skill:** _Participate with peer_

Initials	Material/Activity	Support		Acq. +/✓/–	Sample Student Response/Notes	Maint. +/✓/–
HC	Pretend kitchen, structured play	(F) / P	(Ph) V Vs G I	✓	Put plates on table, stirred pot with spoon	+
HC	Pretend kitchen, structured play	(F) / P	(Ph) V Vs G I	–	(Losing interest, parallel play instead)	+
LR	Outside time, superheroes	(F) / P	Ph V Vs (G) I	–	Followed peer to slide, then distracted	+
		F / P	Ph V Vs G I			
SUMMARY	Most frequent level of response:	–		Most frequent support level:		Partial Verbal

Goal/Curriculum Area: _Count, recognize numerals, find quantities from 1–20._

Maintenance Skill: _Recognition_   **Acquisition Skill:** _Up to 20 and rote counting to 10_

Initials	Material/Activity	Support		Acq. +/✓/–	Sample Student Response/Notes	Maint. +/✓/–
LR	Snack; pretzels	F / (P)	Ph (V) Vs G I	✓	Counted 16 pretzels, motivated by my turns	+
JS	Art time	(F) / P	Ph V (Vs) G I	✓	Counted 17 shakes of glitter, w/number line	+
JS	Art time	(F) / P	Ph (V) Vs G I	✓	Chose bin with 15 crayons	+
HC	Circle time	F / (P)	Ph V (Vs) G I	+	Recognized 1–20 on calendar	+
SUMMARY	Most frequent level of response:	✓		Most frequent support level:		Partial Verbal or Visual

Goal/Curriculum Area: _____

Maintenance Skill: _____   **Acquisition Skill:**

Initials	Material/Activity	Support		Acq. +/✓/–	Sample Student Response/Notes	Maint. +/✓/–
		F / P	Ph V Vs G I			
		F / P	Ph V Vs G I			
		F / P	Ph V Vs G I			
		F / P	Ph V Vs G I			
SUMMARY	Most frequent level of response:			Most frequent support level:		

transferred the information by entering a "+/FV" for the date 10/24. The teacher took data on Julia's requesting goal during a reading activity and a play activity. Julia received a "+/FV" rating and a "✓/PV" rating during the reading activity. During the play activity, Julia received a "✓/FV" rating and a "+/FV" rating. Julia's most frequent level of response is recorded as a "+," as there were two "+" and two "✓," so the best level is recorded. The most frequent support level required is recorded as "FV," because Julia required full verbal support to respond on three out of four data recordings. Data on several other benchmarks are shown in this form for illustrative purposes and have not been transferred to the example of _Handout 7: CPRT Goal Summary_ (see _Figure 6.7_), but note the Summary scores for each goal to understand how these scores were calculated.

here; if the goal requires 10 independent responses, then the number of independent responses should be recorded here). It is important to note that the number of trials correct listed at the top section of each goal only refers to the number of acquisition trials the student responded to at the specified level of support. No maintenance skills, and no acquisition skills that the student needed more support to complete, should be counted as correct when you are computing the student's performance. The score should then be transferred to *Handout 7: CPRT Goal Summary*. A completed example of the *CPRT Data Record: Structured* form is shown in *Figure 6.10*.

CPRT Group Data Records

When you are using CPRT with a group of students, it may be helpful to use a data form designed for collecting data on multiple students at once. Two data forms are included in the manual for this purpose— *Handout 11: CPRT Group Data Record: Tally*, and *Handout 12: CPRT Group Data Record: Rating*. Either the adult conducting the activity, or another teacher or paraprofessional who is supporting the group activity, can record data on either of these forms. Though these forms may not permit you to collect as detailed information as the individual *CPRT Data Record* forms do, both group methods specified here are valuable for keeping general records of student responsiveness and performance during group activities in your classroom.

CPRT GROUP DATA RECORD: TALLY

Handout 11: CPRT Group Data Record: Tally allows you to track progress for several students on different, but essentially similar, benchmarks during one classroom activity. List the names of the students who are participating in the activity down the left-hand side of the form, and identify and list goal areas to target with the students across the top. Then specify the benchmark or level of that goal for each student. For example, the goal area specified in the top row may be "Spontaneous requests." The level for one student may be "Word approximations," while another student is working on "Two-word phrases." During the activity, keep a tally of how many independent and prompted responses each student makes in each goal area (as well as missed opportunities to respond, if appropriate), and record the tallies in the spaces indicated. Taking data during group CPRT interactions can be difficult to manage at first, so it may be helpful to take data on one student at a time and rotate through the group over the course of the activity.

Only information on goals measuring the frequency of particular behavior (e.g., specifying the student will use a spontaneous request a certain number of times throughout the day) can be transferred to *Handout 7: CPRT Goal Summary* form from *Handout 11: CPRT Group Data Record: Tally*. Data on goals measuring behavior in other ways will need to be taken on individual *CPRT Data Record* forms in order to track student progress accurately. A completed example of the *CPRT Group Data Record: Tally* form is shown in *Figure 6.11*.

CPRT GROUP DATA RECORD: RATING

Handout 12: CPRT Group Data Record: Rating is similar to the *CPRT Group Data Record: Tally* form, except that instead of tracking the frequency of particular student behaviors, you rate your students' performance on each goal area from 1 to 5. This can be done every few minutes throughout the activity. To use this form, list the names of the students who are participating in the activity down the left-hand side of the form, and identify and list goal areas to target with

HANDOUT 10	**CPRT Data Record: Structured**	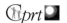

Student: **Julia**   Date: **11/4**

To use this data record, take data on each individual trial in which you present an opportunity to respond to your student. Enter goals to be addressed with CPRT in the spaces provided, and define maintenance and acquisition skills for each goal. In each trial column, indicate whether you targeted a maintenance or acquisition skill, the child's response, and the support level used (if any; you may also just make a mark in the support box if you are not gathering support-type information). At the end of the session, calculate the total number or percent of acquisition trials in which the child responded correctly and independently (number of acquisition trials correct and independent/total number of acquisition trials), depending on what is being measured. Enter this information at the top of each box. Use the Comments section to indicate any important information about that particular goal, such as difficulty with maintenance skills or helpful materials. Use the General Notes section to indicate overall impressions from the session, including student affect, motivation level, and inappropriate behaviors.

Because you will be using CPRT in the context of play and other semistructured activities, intensive trial-by-trial data collection can inhibit the natural flow of interaction between you and your student. To resolve this issue, try completing three to four trials, then allowing the child extended access to the activity materials while you record the data.

Response:
+: Correct response
Att: Attempt toward correct response
−: Incorrect response
NR: No response

Support Level:
F: Full or **P:** Partial

Support Type:
Ph: Physical, **V:** Verbal, **Vs:** Visual, **G:** Gestural

Teacher: **JS**	Goal: **Labels for requests w/partial verbal model**	Acquisition Trials Correct (% or #): **6/11**

Acquisition Skill: **baby, spoon, cookie**

Maintenance Skill: **bottle, spoon, book, juice**

Trial	1	2	3	4	5	6	7	8	9	10	11	12	13	14	15	16	17	18	19	20
Target	(M)/A	M/(A)	M/(A)	(M)/A	M/(A)	(M)/A	M/(A)	M/(A)	(M)/A	M/(A)	M/(A)	(M)/A	M/(A)	(M)/A	M/(A)	(M)/A	M/(A)	(M)/A	M/(A)	M/A
Response	(+)	(+)	(Att)	(NR)	(+)	(+)	(+)	(+)	(+)	(Att)	(NR)	(+)	(Att)	(+)	(+)	(−)	(+)	(Att)	(+)	+
Prompt		PV			PV		FV	PV					PV		PV				PV	

Comments:
Partial verbal model = providing initial sound
Trouble with juice

Teacher: **JS**	Goal: **5 rep. play actions**	Acquisition Trials Correct (% or #): **3/7**

Acquisition Skill: **2- or 3-step seq., novel actions**

Maintenance Skill: **1-step seq., carrying baby**

Trial	1	2	3	4	5	6	7	8	9	10	11	12	13	14	15	16	17	18	19	20
Target	(M)/A	(M)/A	M/(A)	(M)/A	M/(A)	(M)/A	M/(A)	(M)/A	(M)/A	(M)/A	M/(A)	(M)/A	M/(A)	M/(A)	(M)/A	M/(A)	M/A	M/A	M/A	M/A
Response	(+)	(+)	(NR)	(+)	(Att)	(+)	(Att)	(+)	(NR)	(+)	(+)	(+)	(+)	(+)	(+)	(+)	+	+	+	+
Prompt				FG			FG				FG									

Comments:
Full gestural = model of play action sequence
Likes washing baby, sleeping baby, and baby with stroller

(cont.)

FIGURE 6.10. Completed Example of *Handout 10: CPRT Data Record: Structured*. On this form, Julia's teacher and paraprofessionals in her classroom have recorded detailed data on three of Julia's goals. In the trials regarding Julia's ability to label novel items, teachers recorded a total of 19 trials. Eight of these trials were maintenance tasks, and on five of the maintenance trials Julia responded correctly. You can see that on Trial 4 she did not respond, on Trial 16 she was incorrect, and on Trial 18 she was reinforced for an attempt. In this interaction, the teacher presented 11 acquisition trials. To these acquisition cues, Julia responded correctly and independently once (Trial 17); she responded with the support of a partial verbal model five times (Trials 2, 5, 8, 15, and 19); she responded correctly when provided with a full verbal model once (Trial 7); the teacher reinforced her attempt three times (Trials 3, 10, and 13); and once Julia did not respond (Trial 11). Because Julia's current benchmark specifies that she request items after a partial verbal model, only responses in which she demonstrated the skill at this level of support or less were counted as correct. Therefore, in this example, she received a 6/11 (1 response with no prompt and 5 with a partial verbal prompt out of a total of 11 acquisition trials presented). Notice how this 6/11 was transferred to *Handout 7: CPRT Goal Summary* (see *Figure 6.7*) during Period 1 for the second benchmark (date 11/4).

Teacher: **Ms. Holly**	Goal: **Numerals 1–20**										Acquisition Trials Correct (% or #): **1/4 = 25%**								
Acquisition Skill: **11–20**																			
Maintenance Skill: **1–10**																			

Trial	1	2	3	4	5	6	7	8	9	10	11	12	13	14	15	16	17	18	19	20
Target	Ⓜ	Ⓜ	Ⓜ	M	Ⓜ	Ⓜ	M	M	Ⓜ	Ⓜ	M	Ⓜ	Ⓜ	M	M	M	M	M	M	M
	A	A	A	Ⓐ	A	A	Ⓐ	Ⓐ	A	A	Ⓐ	A	A	A	A	A	A	A	A	A
Response	+	⊕	⊕	+	⊕	⊕	+	⊕	⊕	+	+	⊕	⊕	+	+	+	+	+	+	+
	Att	Att	Att	ⒶⓉⓉ	Att	Att	Att	Att	Att	Att	ⒶⓉⓉ	Att	Att	Att	Att	Att	Att	Att	Att	Att
	−	−	−	−	−	−	−	−	−	−	−	−	−	−	−	−	−	−	−	−
	ⓃⓇ	NR	NR	NR	NR	NR	ⓃⓇ	NR	NR	ⓃⓇ	NR	NR	NR	NR	NR	NR	NR	NR	NR	NR
Prompt		Ph		PV								FV								

Comments:
Motivated to count items for eating
Putting finger on item to encourage continued counting = physical prompt

FIGURE 6.10. *(cont.)*

the students across the top. Then specify the benchmark or level of that goal for each student. During the activity, pause briefly after a few minutes and circle a rating for each student for each skill, using the scale provided on the form (1 = no response/maximal prompting required at all opportunities, 5 = primarily independent responses). At the end of the activity, circle a score to reflect each student's motivation level through the majority of the activity. It may be helpful to rotate around the group and rate all goals for one student during each pause, rather than attempting to complete every rating at each opportunity. Alternatively, you could rotate through the goals and rate each student on a single skill during one pause, and move to the next goal at the next opportunity.

Though *Handout 12: CPRT Group Data Record: Rating* only collects general information about the level of student response, it is useful to assess generalization of skills. For example, if a student is consistently receiving a rating of 5 for making comments to peers in one activity, but a rating of 2 in another activity, it may be necessary to work with this student on generalizing this skill to new settings. Ratings from this sheet cannot be transferred to *Handout 7: CPRT Goal Summary*, because it is a general evaluation of level of response rather than a form for specific measurement

of behavior. A completed example of the *CPRT Group Data Record: Rating* form is shown in *Figure 6.12*.

Practice Makes Perfect

This collection of forms is intended to be a guide for streamlining your CPRT data collection process. Taking data during instruction is a learned skill, and it is especially difficult in a group setting. It may be necessary to practice often before you feel at ease conducting activities (especially group activities) while collecting information on your students. Also, remember that data on student skills are only useful to the extent that they are used to plan instruction—don't just take data, use them!

 Reproducible blank copies of all the data collection and planning forms are provided in *Part IV*.

Using CPRT to Encourage Generalization

Poor generalization of skills is a common problem for students with autism. This means that a student who can use certain skills under one set of circumstances is not

CPRT Group Data Record: Tally

Activity: __Art time__   Teacher: __Ms. Smith__   Date: __10/12/09__

This sheet allows you to keep data during group instruction. Though not all students have identical goals, grouping those with similar goals will help you use this form.

Before the activity begins: Write several goals relevant to the activity across the top of the grid below, and list the participating students on the left. Make a note of the current acquisition skill for each student in each column. **During the activity:** Record data by tallying the number of times each student demonstrates the skill independently (Ind) and with prompting (Pmt). Taking data while teaching a group of students is a learned skill, but with practice it is possible to conduct group instruction while tracking student responses. To start, you may want to record data on one student for an interval of time and then switch to a second student, and so forth, or select one or two students to track each day, so that data collection remains manageable.

Student	Goal/Behavior: *Verbally request desired items*	Goal/Behavior: *Counting*	Goal/Behavior: *Color identification*	Goal/Behavior: *Turn taking*	Motivation
Michelle	Skill: **1-word appx.** Ind: III Pmt: IIII Miss Opp: I	Skill: **Rote to 5** Ind: IIII Pmt: IIII Miss Opp:	Skill: **Receptive ident.** Ind: I Pmt: IIII Miss Opp: II	Skill: **Indicate desire** Ind: II Pmt: IIII I Miss Opp:	1 2 ③ 4 5
Bryan	Skill: **1-2 words** Ind: III Pmt: II Miss Opp:	Skill: **Match up to 5** Ind: IIII I Pmt: Miss Opp:	Skill: **Expressive label** Ind: II Pmt: IIII II Miss Opp: II	Skill: **Facilitated turn** Ind: IIII Pmt: II Miss Opp:	1 2 ③ 4 5
Kalea	Skill: **2- or 3-wd. phrase** Ind: III Pmt: IIII Miss Opp: III	Skill: **N/A** Ind: Pmt: Miss Opp:	Skill: **N/A** Ind: Pmt: Miss Opp:	Skill: **Initiate turns** Ind: III Pmt: IIII I Miss Opp: III	1 ② 3 4 5
Joshua	Skill: **1-2 words** Ind: IIII Pmt: II Miss Opp: I	Skill: **Rote to 5** Ind: I Pmt: II Miss Opp: I	Skill: **Receptive ident.** Ind: IIII Pmt: I Miss Opp:	Skill: **N/A** Ind: Pmt: Miss Opp:	1 2 3 ④ 5

FIGURE 6.11. Completed Example of *Handout 11: CPRT Group Data Record: Tally.* On this form, Ms. Smith has taken data on a group of four students during an art activity. She has identified four goal areas (requests, counting, color identification, and turn taking) that are relevant to all or some of these students. Notice that if a goal is not relevant for a particular child, the teacher has simply entered N/A in the appropriate space (e.g., Kalea is not currently working on color identification, so no goal is entered for her in this column). If Kalea has a goal to initiate 5 turns with a peer during an activity, the teacher may transfer a 3 from this data sheet to *Handout 7: CPRT Goal Summary* (see *Figure 6.7*), as this is the number of times Kalea was able to use this skill independently according to the data.

CPRT Group Data Record: Rating

Activity: **Art time** Teacher: **Ms. Smith** Date: **10/12/04**

This sheet allows you to keep data during group instruction. Though not all students have identical goals, grouping those with similar goals will help you use this form.

Before the activity begins: Write several goals relevant to the activity across the top of the grid below, and list the participating students on the left. Make a note of the current acquisition skill for each student in each column. **During the activity:** Record data by rating each student's performance of the acquisition skill from 1 to 5 at three points during the activity. Use the rating scale below. It may be easiest to set a timer for one-third the planned length of the activity and record data when the timer sounds. Alternatively, it may be helpful to rate one student in all areas every few minutes, so that data collection remains manageable. At the end, rate each student's motivation from 1 to 5. To start, you may want to record data on one student for an interval of time and then switch to a second student, and so forth, or select one or two students to track each day, so that data collection remains manageable.

1: No response/maximal prompting required at all opportunities
2: Maximal prompting required at most opportunities; no independent responses
3: Some prompting required at most opportunities; sporadic independent responses
4: Some independent responses (at least 50%); some prompted responses
5: Primarily independent responses (more than 75% of responses independent)

Student	Goal: Verbally request desired items	Goal: Counting	Goal: Color identification	Goal: Turn taking	Motivation
Michelle	Skill: **1-word appx.** — Rating: 1 2 3 ④ 5 / 1 2 3 ④ 5 / 1 2 ③ 4 5	Skill: **Rote to 5** — Rating: 1 2 3 4 ⑤ / 1 2 3 4 ⑤ / 1 2 3 4 ⑤	Skill: **Receptive ident.** — Rating: 1 2 ③ 4 5 / 1 2 ③ 4 5 / 1 2 3 ④ 5	Skill: **Indicate desire** — Rating: 1 2 3 ④ 5 / 1 2 3 4 5 / 1 2 3 ④ 5	1 2 3 ④ 5
Bryan	Skill: **1-2 words** — Rating: 1 2 ③ 4 5 / 1 ② 3 4 5 / 1 2 ③ 4 5	Skill: **Match up to 5** — Rating: 1 ② 3 4 5 / 1 ② 3 4 5 / 1 2 3 ④ 5	Skill: **Expressive label** — Rating: 1 2 3 ④ 5 / 1 2 ③ 4 5 / 1 2 3 ④ 5	Skill: **Facilitated turn** — Rating: 1 2 3 ④ 5 / 1 2 ③ 4 ⑤ / 1 2 ③ 4 5	1 2 ③ 4 5
Kalea	Skill: **2- or 3-word phrase** — Rating: 1 ② 3 4 5 / 1 ② 3 4 5 / 1 2 3 4 5	Skill: **N/A**	Skill: **N/A**	Skill: **Initiate turns** — Rating: 1 ② 3 4 5 / 1 ② 3 4 5 / 1 ② 3 4 5	1 ② 3 4 5
Joshua	Skill: **1-2 words** — Rating: 1 2 3 4 5 / 1 ② 3 4 5 / 1 ② 3 4 5	Skill: **Rote to 5** — Rating: 1 2 ③ 4 5 / 1 2 3 4 5 / 1 ② 3 4 5	Skill: **Receptive ident.** — Rating: 1 2 ③ 4 5 / 1 2 ③ 4 5 / 1 2 ③ 4 5	Skill: **N/A**	1 ② 3 4 5

FIGURE 6.12. Completed Example of *Handout 12: CPRT Group Data Record: Rating.* This form covers the same activity and student goals as *Handout 11: CPRT Group Data Record: Tally.* However, here the teacher has rated student performance in each area on the 1–5 scale at several time points during the activity. You can see that Michelle was fairly motivated throughout the activity (motivation rating = 4) and received mostly 3's, 4's, and 5's for her skills, Kalea was less motivated (motivation rating = 2) and received primarily 2's and 3's. This may be an indication to the teacher to find alternative ways to motivate Kalea during art time.

able to use the same skills under different conditions. For example, when you say, "Good morning, John, how are you?", John can correctly respond, "I'm fine, Ms. Nelson. How are you?" However, when the new speech therapist, Mr. Lui, says, "Morning, John! How's it going?" as they pass each other in the hallway, John looks past him and says nothing. John is not able to generalize the skill of responding to a greeting. If a student does not generalize what he has learned, the skill is not truly useful.

CPRT is conducive to promoting generalization of skills, because it is a naturalistic intervention.

CPRT incorporates strategies that promote generalization. Still, there are additional factors that can enhance generalization and contribute to the overall success of a CPRT program.

- Use CPRT with varied teachers, settings, and materials, to increase the likelihood that your student will respond to CPRT under a wide variety of circumstances.
  - Have multiple adults implement CPRT with your students (e.g., teacher, paraprofessional, parents, speech therapist, occupational therapist).
  - Use CPRT in multiple activities and settings throughout the day (e.g., circle time, snack time, playground, lunchroom).
  - Implement CPRT with varied materials (e.g., toys, academic materials, snacks).
- Use teaching materials that interest the student and are readily available in the environment. Ensuring student motivation will maximize learning.
  - Use developmentally appropriate materials to encourage play skills and keep the student motivated.

  - Materials should be well organized and easy to access (or visible and easy to request).
  - When choosing materials, consider findings from *Handout 3: Gathering Information* and the structured preference assessments (*Handouts 4–5*). Or, if you don't have this information available, observe the student in unstructured play and note the student's reaction when you take a toy away. If the student reacts strongly, it indicates a preference for the toy. Notice what non-toy objects the student enjoys as well.
- Anticipate when CPRT can be used throughout the day.
  - Develop routines and use CPRT to require your student to request the next step (e.g., put on shoes and get your student's backpack, then wait for her to initiate a request to go to the car or bus).
  - Intentionally remove important pieces of an activity to encourage communication (during snack time, put out a cup without juice and wait for your student to request juice; get paper out for coloring, but "forget" the crayons).
  - Use environmental arrangement to encourage communication (place favorite toys or foods out of the student's reach; use containers that are clear but difficult to open).

Using the strategies above to promote students' generalization will help them use and maintain their skills over time. *Handout 13: CPRT Generalization Probe* (available in *Part IV*) allows you to measure the generalization of specific student skills. Use this worksheet and your observations to ensure your students consistently generalize the new skills they learn. A completed example of the *CPRT Generalization Probe* form is shown in *Figure 6.13*.

CPRT Generalization Probe   *Cprt*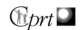

Student: **Amir**

Goal Domain: **Expressive; requesting**   Benchmark: **3- to 5-word phrases to request assistance**

To ensure that a skill target is functional for your student, you must know if he/she can use this skill in a variety of circumstances. Identify three different materials, settings, and teachers for the purpose of probing the skill listed above. The materials you choose should be highly preferred by the student.

Materials/Activity: 1. Putting straw in juice box
                         2. Opening containers
                         3. Accessing out-of-reach items

Setting: 1. Snack table
              2. Art table
              3. Play area

Partner: 1. Ms. Smith
              2. Ms. Holly
              3. Mr. Jack

Indicate the date and the circumstances in which you will probe the skill. Circle the number that corresponds with the specific materials, setting, or teacher listed above. Circle the student's response to the probed skill target as Correct (C), Incorrect (I), or No Response (NR).

Date	Materials			Setting			Teacher			Student Response		
6/5/09	(1)	2	3	(1)	2	3	1	2	(3)	(C)	I	NR
6/6/09	1	(2)	3	1	2	(3)	1	(2)	3	C	I	(NR)
6/6/09	1	(2)	3	1	(2)	3	1	2	(3)	(C)	I	NR
6/7/09	(1)	2	3	(1)	2	3	(1)	2	3	C	(I)	NR
6/9/09	1	2	(3)	1	(2)	3	1	(2)	3	C	I	(NR)
6/10/09	1	2	(3)	1	2	(3)	1	2	(3)	C	(I)	NR
6/13/09	1	(2)	3	(1)	2	3	(1)	2	3	(C)	I	NR
6/13/09	1	(2)	3	1	2	(3)	(1)	2	3	(C)	I	NR
6/14/09	(1)	2	3	(1)	2	3	1	(2)	3	C	(I)	NR
6/14/09	1	(2)	3	1	2	(3)	1	2	(3)	(C)	I	NR
6/14/09	1	(2)	3	1	(2)	3	(1)	2	3	(C)	I	NR
	1	2	3	1	2	3	1	2	3	C	I	NR
	1	2	3	1	2	3	1	2	3	C	I	NR
	1	2	3	1	2	3	1	2	3	C	I	NR
	1	2	3	1	2	3	1	2	3	C	I	NR
Total	*3*	*6*	*2*	*4*	*3*	*4*	*4*	*3*	*4*	*6*	*3*	*2*

Summary: **Continue goal. Amir is having difficulty requesting assistance from Ms. Holly. Review prompting techniques from others to promote independence with Ms. Holly.**

FIGURE 6.13. Completed Example of *Handout 13: CPRT Generalization Probe.* On this form, Amir's teacher has collected information on his ability to use 3- to 5-word requests for assistance across several activities, settings, and partners. After reviewing the form, she notices that Amir is not consistently using the skill with one teacher, Ms. Holly. She makes a note to review prompting techniques with Ms. Holly, as it is possible that Ms. Holly is providing too much support to Amir, and thus he is having difficulty using the skill independently with her.

Troubleshooting

This section highlights some common questions from teachers who use CPRT.

What if my student will not pay attention?

- Begin by expecting only brief periods of attention; then slowly increase your expectations as your student is successful.
- Use the *Hierarchy of Opportunities to Respond* (please see *Chapter 2, Table 2.1*) to provide your student added assistance. The student may need more structured opportunities (verbal model, instruction) before moving to more advanced types of opportunities (expectant waiting, situational, etc.).
- Be sure you are engaging your student with an appropriate level of affect and animation.
- Be sure you are using motivating materials, activities, or topics.

What if my student moves quickly between activities and will not stay with one activity?

Consider a few possible factors:

- Decide whether the tasks are too demanding. Even with an activity that a student enjoys, too many acquisition tasks in a row or too little reinforcement can cause the student to become frustrated. Try increasing maintenance tasks, increasing the level of rewards, and making sure the interaction is fun and interesting.
- If a student simply has a short attention span, you can make sure that he has to indicate "all done" and ask for the next activity. Sometimes simply having to make a request to end a task keeps a student with that task longer.
- Try having the student do it "one more time" or stay "one more minute" before moving to the next activity. This can help you complete activities with a group of students and can increase students' attention to tasks.

What if my student is overly focused on one activity?

- If a student becomes extremely focused on one activity and resists switching to new activities or terminating play, you can limit the activities from which she chooses. For example, if your student becomes very agitated when she has to leave the computer, you can use a visual timer and icon to help her anticipate when computer time will be over, but you may also decide not to present the computer as one of the choices.
- Items of high focus may also be very motivating for students; therefore, they can often be incorporated into activities to be used as rewards.
- Students can be taught to use items of high focus (or topics of interest) more appropriately.

What if my student responds inappropriately more often than making attempts or responding correctly?

- Change the teaching approach, prompt level, and expectations. Perhaps the student is having a difficult day, he does not feel well, or something in the teaching environment is distracting and the student needs more support.
- Try to increase the student's motivation by allowing the student to choose new activities or materials.
- Increase reinforcement by rewarding more attempts.
- Provide more maintenance tasks.

What if my staff and I are having difficulty gaining control of reinforcing items?

- Gather preferred objects in advance, and block the student's access to the preferred object or activity until a response occurs. For example, John has chosen to play with an animal puzzle and starts to put the zebra piece into the puzzle. You may cover the spot for the zebra on the puzzle until he says, "Put in," or "Zebra" (whatever his current language goal is). When John provides an appropriate response, he is allowed to put in the puzzle piece.

- Take a turn to gain control of the materials.
- Cover the materials with a cloth or put the materials in a box, so that only you have access to them.

Where do I begin if my student is not using verbal communication?

- Many students who have a young chronological or developmental age benefit from CPRT. If your student does not use verbal communication yet, you can focus on other communication skills.
- Target eye contact, reaching, pointing, gestures, or sign language by making the student's access to desired items contingent on her use of one of these skills.
- A picture communication system may also be appropriate for students with limited language.

What if my student is not motivated?

- Update the student's preference assessment to find effective reinforcers.
- Look more creatively at what the student is doing during his free time, and incorporate these materials or activities into specific lessons.
- Adjust the reinforcement value of available materials by limiting access to favorite toys, activities, and foods.
- If your student is rarely successful at earning reinforcers, this may decrease motivation. It may be helpful to increase the number of maintenance tasks you provide and to reward attempts more often.
- Be sure you are taking very brief turns and adjusting your animation level to meet your student's needs.

What if my student demonstrates challenging behavior when I am using CPRT?

The first step is to assess the antecedents:

- Remember not to place demands on your student every time you come near. If you do, your student may be anticipating the demand. Be sure to spend some time having fun with your student. At times, simply approach your student and say hello or give her a high five, so that she does not expect a demand from you all the time.
- Increase the number of maintenance tasks or increase the number of attempts you are rewarding. Presenting difficult tasks all the time can lead to frustration. A frustrated student is more likely to engage in problem behaviors.
- Check that your cues and expectations are developmentally appropriate. Be sure the language you are using to give instructions is at a level your student can understand. Be sure the skill you are expecting is at or just above your student's developmental level.
- Make sure the tasks are motivating. Be sure that your student has a choice of activity, or that some aspect of the activity has been selected to increase motivation. Try to include something the student enjoys within the activity.

Next, assess the consequences you are providing.

- Be sure that you are not accidentally rewarding inappropriate behaviors. Many students are reinforced by any form of attention. You may feel as if you are reprimanding a student, but the attention itself may be rewarding. Frustrated facial expressions or exasperated sighs can be reinforcing. Try to remain calm and quiet during inappropriate behaviors, keeping students safe with as little attention as possible.
- Remember not to decrease demands contingent upon the inappropriate behaviors. Sometimes students engage in inappropriate behavior because it is a good way to avoid doing something. Be sure that if you present your student with a task, she needs to respond appropriately in order to receive a reward or terminate the activity. Try to offer other ways to ask for a break (e.g., a break card).
- Provide enough reinforcement. Be sure you are rewarding appropriate behavior and task completion with something the stu-

dent enjoys. You may need to increase the frequency of the rewards for difficult or nonpreferred tasks.

What if my student has restricted play interests or does not like toys?

- Use your student's restricted interests as reinforcers for appropriate play.
- Use your turns strategically, modeling new play actions.
- Use fun animation that will engage your student and keep his attention.
- Incorporate novel play with familiar toy play by sometimes modeling a familiar action to keep the student's interest, and at other times doing something new.

What if my student will only play with one toy?

- If this is the case, start with that toy. Identify other skills to teach with the same toy. For example, if she will only play with a pinwheel and wants to roll it on her arm, have her blow the wheel with her mouth, ask a friend to blow, hold it in front of a fan, draw a pinwheel, pretend it's a flower, and so on. Next, add other toys/objects to the play by having the pinwheel ride on a dump truck, using the pinwheel as a magic wand for a magician's costume, or pretending it is a spoon to mix cake batter. Once new actions and objects are incorporated, increase the number of steps the student needs to complete before getting free access to the pinwheel.
- Limit the student's choices, and ensure that sometimes the preferred toy is not available. Provide choices of other activities instead. It is important that your student learn to play appropriately with the preferred toy, so you will want to work with it at times, but it is acceptable to provide other choices and take the preferred toy out of the mix sometimes as well.

What toys should I use to encourage play?

- Choose toys that your student enjoys, and items that will encourage play at the appropriate developmental level.

- To begin, observe the student in free play, to see what he chooses when left on his own. This is often a good place to start.
- When you take the toy away, watch to see if the student becomes upset or tries to keep the toy. This is a good indication that the toy is a good reinforcer.
- Determine which non-toy objects the student enjoys. These can be incorporated into play and can also be used for symbolic play.
- It is also important to incorporate toys that other students in your class enjoy. You want to teach play that is developmentally appropriate; however, if it is possible to use toys and materials that are age-appropriate, this can help with social acceptance. For example, teaching symbolic play with cars and action figures rather than with *Sesame Street* characters would be helpful for a second grader.

What if my student is avoidant of peers?

- Begin by simply having your student be near other students. You may need to begin with only one other student who is 3 feet away and gradually decrease the distance between the students.
- Introduce an activity based on the interests of your student, and then use your level of excitement to naturally attract the attention of other students too. Be animated and enthusiastic to encourage others to join you and maintain proximity to the student with autism.

How can my student play with peers if she does not talk?

- Use simple forms of interaction (taking turns with a ball, playing near friends, sharing a tub of paint, collecting papers, etc.).
- Focus on ways to interact with others that do not require language. For example, playing a game of tag requires interaction but little language.

How can I encourage interaction if my student is bright but very socially awkward?

- Begin by trying to figure out whether your student may be able to change some simple things to become more socially acceptable to peers.

- Try working on concrete goals, such as maintaining physical space and appropriate tone of voice (or whatever your student needs). Reward your student for using appropriate vocal tone, choosing good conversation topics, and maintaining eye contact.
- Incorporate other strategies, such as video modeling and social stories, to assist your student with understanding complex social interactions.
- Be sure you are being spontaneous in the way you are prompting and modeling social interactions, so that rote behavior will be reduced.

What if there is no natural or direct reinforcer for the task I am teaching?

- This may be your first reaction to many tasks, especially academic ones. However, many tasks can be adapted to include a natural reward. This will increase your student's motivation to engage in the activity, which should enhance learning and reduce behavior issues.
- Incorporate something of interest to your student into the activity.
- Find specific activities that can occur across various lessons to motivate your student. For example, a student may enjoy collecting materials or assignment from the class upon completion of his own work, or selecting a different-colored pencil after finishing each math problem.
- Of course, there will be things your student needs to learn that will require indi-

rect rewards. Those skills should be taught using another technique.

What if my student has to learn a skill and cannot be given a choice?

It is true that there are some skills students need to learn, whether they want to or not.

- Try to incorporate some sort of choice into the activity itself. For example, perhaps your student can choose where to sit or which materials to use within the activity itself. There may be the opportunity to choose whose turn it will be next or when to leave the activity.
- Of course, in these cases you are not following your student's lead, but at least you are giving some opportunity for choice making.
- In some cases, you may be able to follow your student's lead and still work on a specific goal. For example, almost any activity your student does could involve some counting or color identification.

 For more information on video modeling, see *Video Modeling: A Visual Teaching Method for Children with Autism* by Lisa Neumann (2004); *www.asatonline.org/ intervention/treatments/video.htm*; *www.modelmekids.com/video- modeling.html*; and *www. watchmelearn.com*. For information on social stories, see *The New Social Story Book* by Carol Gray (2010); *www.thegraycenter.com*.

PART III

Resources
and Support

CHAPTER 7

Training Paraprofessionals

CHAPTER OVERVIEW

Teachers are typically responsible for training paraprofessional educators in specific teaching strategies. This chapter outlines strategies for training your staff, and the procedures for assessing implementation of CPRT.

The following sections are included:

The Training Process
    Step 1: Have the Paraprofessional View Instructional Videos
    Step 2: Model CPRT
    Step 3: Observe, Assess, and Provide Feedback
    Step 4: Refer the Paraprofessional to the *CPRT Component Summary Sheets*

Assessing Implementation of CPRT
    Using the *CPRT Assessment* and *CPRT Feedback*

Maintaining and Improving Skills

This chapter has a corresponding training lecture on the DVD accompanying this manual (*CPRT Session 5: Educating Paraprofessionals and Parents about CPRT*).

When paraprofessional educators join your classroom team, you are likely to be responsible for training them in the strategies you use to educate your students. This chapter provides you with resources for training the paraprofessionals in your classroom to use CPRT and assessing their implementation of the components. Also, there are suggested resources for improving a paraprofessional's understanding of autism and related disorders, as well as of general behavioral management strategies. Four training lectures (each lasting 10–15 minutes) are included on the DVD accompanying this manual. The lectures are designed to be viewed independently by your paraprofessionals.

The Training Process

We recommend that you use the following general steps to prepare a paraprofessional to implement CPRT:

1. Have the paraprofessional view the training lecture.

2. Model the CPRT component(s) with students while the paraprofessional observes.

3. Observe the paraprofessional's use of the components, assess implementation, and provide feedback.

4. Refer the paraprofessional to the *CPRT Component Summary Sheets* (see *Part IV, Handouts 21–28*) for a review of each component.

Steps 2–4 are repeated until each of the components has been mastered. Each step is discussed in more detail below.

Step 1: Have the Paraprofessional View Instructional Videos

As noted above, four short training lectures (each lasting 10–15 minutes) provide information on behavioral principles and the components of CPRT. The videos are narrated and include examples of teachers using the techniques. *Session 1: What Is CPRT?* provides a description of how CPRT was developed, as well as of the behavioral foundation for the specific components of CPRT. *Session 2: Antecedent Strategies for CPRT* describes the specific components of CPRT that relate to antecedent strategies. *Session 3: Student Behavior and Consequence Strategies for CPRT* describes how paraprofessionals can better understand their students' behavior, and explains the specific components of CPRT that relate to consequence strategies. *Session 4: CPRT with Groups* gives additional strategies for using CPRT with multiple students at one time. See *Table 7.1* for a description of the behaviors you should model and the resources you can share after paraprofessionals watch each training lecture.

TABLE 7.1. Paraprofessional Training

This table provides a reference for specific components of CPRT addressed by each paraprofessional training lecture and the accompanying CPRT Component Summary Sheets.

Paraprofessional training lecture	Components to model	*CPRT Component Summary Sheets*
Session 1. What Is CPRT?	None	None
Session 2. Antecedent Strategies for CPRT	1. Student attention 2. Clear and appropriate instruction 3. Easy and difficult tasks 4. Shared control 5. Multiple cues	*Handout 21: Component 1: Student Attention* *Handout 22: Component 2: Clear and Appropriate Instruction* *Handout 23: Component 3: Easy and Difficult Tasks* *Handout 24: Component 4: Shared Control* *Handout 25: Component 5: Multiple Cues*
Session 3. Student Behavior and Consequence Strategies for CPRT	6. Direct reinforcement 7. Contingent consequence 8. Reinforcement of attempts	*Handout 26: Component 6: Direct Reinforcement* *Handout 27: Component 7: Contingent Consequence* *Handout 28: Component 8: Reinforcement of Attempts*
Session 4. CPRT with Groups	None	None

Step 2: Model CPRT

Modeling with your students is an excellent way to demonstrate the components of CPRT and make the intervention more relevant and exciting for your staff. You may choose to model CPRT components with one or more students. Choose an activity that is preferred by your students and allows you to easily control the materials. Before you demonstrate CPRT with your students, you may want to complete *Handout 14: CPRT Student Profile* (see *Part IV*). A completed example of this document is provided in *Figure 7.1*. Copy *Handout 14* and make it available to the paraprofessionals in your classroom. Briefly explain the activity to your paraprofessional, and highlight the specific components of CPRT you will be demonstrating. Use *Table 7.1* to determine which components correspond with each training lecture. You will begin with the components that involve setting the stage, and then move through the other components over time. Then take a brief break to comment on the activity and answer any questions. If there isn't enough time to discuss the interaction, ask your paraprofessional to write down questions or comments to be discussed later, as time permits.

Take a few minutes to model the components while working with your students, and try to focus only on the students, withholding any comments to the paraprofessional.

Another helpful step is to make a video recording of yourself modeling CPRT. This can be beneficial for several reasons. First, it may reduce any resistance your paraprofessional may have to being video-recorded. Second, you can use the video-recorded session to show parents or other classroom staff how CPRT works. Finally, observing yourself working with students can help you improve your own use of CPRT.

Step 3: Observe, Assess, and Provide Feedback

Observe the paraprofessional's use of CPRT components, assess implementation, and provide feedback. Research shows that observing, assessing, and providing feedback to staff members individually helps to improve their skills. This can be difficult, however! If you have more than one paraprofessional, you may feel that there is not enough time to work with each person individually. Or you may be uncomfortable tell-

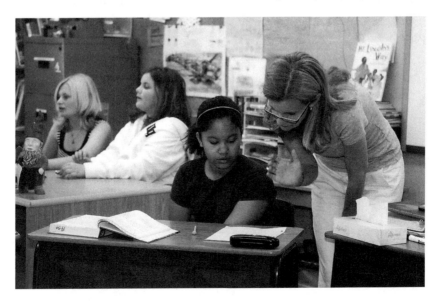

CPRT Student Profile

Student: **Julia**

This form is designed to facilitate communication about a student's preferences and current ability level. Update progress and preferences regularly (weekly is suggested), and share this document with your team. Use the *CPRT Data Record* forms to gather information to complete this profile.

Benchmark/Goal: Label 5–10 new words per month; use words in 2 settings w/2 people.			
Date	**Acquisition**	**Maintenance**	**Preferences**
9/12/08	Bottle, spoon, book Try labels @ lunch (*hotdog, juice, apple*)	Car, ball, baby, phone, cookie	Apple juice, hotdogs, using markers, dinosaurs, pretending to feed doll
9/19/08	Bottle, spoon, marker, hotdog, apple, grapes	Car, ball, baby, phone, book, cookie, juice, "ah" for *apple*	Likes Strawberry Shortcake, apple juice, hotdogs (have mustard for dipping), markers
9/26/08			
10/2/08			

Benchmark/Goal: Perform new representational play actions.			
9/12/08	Bathing baby, putting baby to sleep, setting up picnic	Carrying baby, talking on toy phone, eating pretend food herself	Likes Strawberry Shortcake doll, rocking the cradle. Upset if peer takes blanket.
9/19/08	Bathing baby, setting up picnic, feeding baby with spoon	Carrying baby, eating pretend food herself, putting baby to sleep	Putting baby to sleep moved to maint.
9/26/08			
10/2/08			

(cont.)

FIGURE 7.1. Completed Example of *Handout 14: CPRT Student Profile.* This form lists a student's goals, the best activities in which to target those goals, and helpful tips and notes about those activities. This is a useful tool for sharing student goal information with your classroom team.

Benchmark/Goal:
Participate in play with a peer.

Date	Acquisition	Maintenance	Preferences
9/12/08	Responding to peer requests, sharing toys/materials	Playing near peer, watching peers play	Likes to follow peers on the playground
9/19/08	Same	Same	Enjoys rolling ball up and down slide with peer
9/26/08			
10/2/08			

Benchmark/Goal:
Count and recognize numerals from 1 to 20.

Date	Acquisition	Maintenance	Preferences
9/12/08	Numerals from 11 to 20, counting independently	Numerals from 1 to 10	Count food items at snack, count gross motor activities (wiggles, jumps, etc.)
9/19/08	Same	Same	No new notes
9/26/08			
10/2/08			

Notes:

FIGURE 7.1. *(cont.)*

ing a paraprofessional where improvement is needed. Before you begin, make sure you help your paraprofessional feel comfortable and competent. Complete *Handout 14: CPRT Student Profile* for each student your paraprofessional will be teaching, or complete the document together before you begin your observation. This will remind your paraprofessional to personalize the use of CPRT so that it matches the developmental level(s) of the student(s) involved.

The first few times your paraprofessional tries to use CPRT, it may be difficult. For this reason, we suggest that you focus on a couple of components at a time, using *Table 7.1* as a guide. Once those are mastered, you can have the paraprofessional try additional components, and finally put them all together. Once you feel that your paraprofessional is using CPRT well, you can use *Handout 15: CPRT Assessment* and *Handout 16: CPRT Feedback* (see *Part IV*) to provide more detailed comments, and to assess use of CPRT over time and with varied students.

Try to provide positive feedback, as well as recommendations for improvement.

Step 4: Refer the Paraprofessional to the *CPRT Component Summary Sheets*

After you discuss your paraprofessional's use of CPRT, you may need to provide a review of components that were not implemented well. To save time, *CPRT Component Summary Sheets* (see *Handouts 21–28*) are included in *Part IV*. Each sheet gives a one-page summary of each component, along with tips or additional examples. They offer a quick review and can save you the time required to explain a specific component again. Choose one or two CPRT components that correspond with the train-

ing lecture and modeling for your paraprofessional to reread and practice before your next observation. This will help to focus the staff member's attention.

These four steps are repeated until your paraprofessional can use each component of CPRT. Staff training is an ongoing process. Continue to focus on one or two components during each observation. Ask the paraprofessional to review relevant information, with a reminder to think about the specific components before starting a new observation. The time it takes to train your paraprofessional will depend on several factors. We have found that many of the CPRT components come naturally to trainees; your paraprofessional may be using several components correctly before you even begin structured training in the intervention. Don't be discouraged if some skills are difficult for an individual to learn, however.

The amount of time you can spend observing and providing feedback, as well as the paraprofessional's prior experience, will affect how quickly the components of CPRT are learned.

Assessing Implementation of CPRT

As discussed in *Chapter 6*, fidelity of implementation is the degree to which an intervention is implemented as it was intended. CPRT has been tested repeatedly and has been shown to help students learn. However, this success has been demonstrated when CPRT is implemented correctly and in its entirety. It is not clear how students will benefit from CPRT if only certain components are used or if the components are not used correctly. For this reason, it is important to help your paraprofessionals learn to use the components of CPRT correctly. To do this, you will need use *Handout 15: CPRT Assessment* (see *Part IV*) to assess implementation of the intervention.

Using the *CPRT Assessment* and *CPRT Feedback* Forms

To complete *Handout 15: CPRT Assessment*, first read the brief instructions on the form and familiarize yourself with the scoring categories. Next, consider which skills are easy (maintenance) and difficult (acquisition) for the student or students participating in the observation. This information will help you evaluate how well the paraprofessional intersperses easy and difficult skills with each student. Now you are ready to observe your paraprofessional for approximately 10 minutes. You may want to start by giving suggestions or answering questions during the first 5 minutes, then observing without commenting for the following 5-minute period. It is helpful to explain what you are doing (e.g., "Now take a few minutes to work with Lucia on your own. I'm not going to say anything, so we can both concentrate more on your interaction with Lucia. When you are finished, we will discuss what happened").

While you observe, you should also complete the *CPRT Assessment* document. Keep track of the number of opportunities the paraprofessional provides to the student, and determine the degree to which each component is used correctly. For example, if your paraprofessional follows the student's choice of activity occasionally, but misses a majority of opportunities, you should score a 2. After making a judgment for each of the components in the first category, "Teacher maximizes child motivation," choose an average summary score. The summary score is designed to be an overall rating for the skills in each category. This will help you to identify general areas of strength

and weakness. To choose the appropriate summary score, average the scores for each of the skills in the category. A rating of 4 means that each component is implemented correctly a majority of the time, with only a few missed opportunities. After you complete the assessment, determine which components were used correctly (a score of 4 or 5) and which components still need improvement (a score of 3 or less).

> To meet the fidelity criteria, or mastery criteria, your paraprofessional should use all the components at a level of 4 or above.

Now you are ready to provide useful, data-based feedback to your paraprofessional. *Handout 16: CPRT Feedback* (see *Part IV*) has been developed to help with this process. When providing feedback, be sure to start with a compliment. It is important to highlight what your paraprofessionals are doing well and to encourage their efforts. Ask the paraprofessional how the interaction felt. You should also suggest areas for improvement and give specific examples of what can be done differently. Ask the paraprofessional if there are any questions about CPRT or using it with a specific student. Take time to answer your paraprofessional's questions thoughtfully. Finally, remind the paraprofessional (and yourself) what went well during the observation. Teaching and learning a new intervention can be tedious, and you both need encouragement for your efforts!

Maintaining and Improving Skills

After the members of classroom staff have learned to use CPRT, we recommend that you help them to maintain their skills through ongoing support and supervision.

We offer several suggestions for continued learning.

- *Practice with multiple students.* If you plan to have staff members use CPRT with multiple students, it is a good idea to have them practice and demonstrate fidelity with each of these students. Because students with autism vary considerably with regard to specific skills, motivation levels, and challenging behaviors, it is likely that a paraprofessional's use of CPRT skills will vary across students.

- *Model CPRT.* Be mindful of situations in which you use CPRT throughout the day. Take a moment to explain how you are using these strategies to fit the needs of a specific student, learning goal, or activity. Your continued positive example will provide ongoing learning opportunities that are tailored to your students and classroom.

- *Provide brief weekly or biweekly updates on student progress, new activities, and materials.* As you continue to train your classroom staff, you may want to introduce regular meetings to update paraprofessionals on student progress and strategies for using CPRT in new situations. If you have little or no time when paraprofessionals are available to meet without students present, consider updating your paraprofessionals individually or creating a brief memo that can be posted or kept in a binder for their review. *Handout 17: Classroom Weekly Memo* (see *Part IV*) can be used to write such a memo. A completed example of this form is provided in *Figure 7.2.* Include in your meeting or memo any skills that have advanced from acquisition to maintenance for each student, new classroom materials or centers that are relevant for CPRT use, and new activities that you will be using to model CPRT throughout the day. These

updates will keep you and your staff well informed, will ensure that you are assessing student progress to inform instruction, and should maximize student learning opportunities.

 You may want to refer your paraprofessionals to other sources for information to supplement what you are able to teach them.

www.autismspeaks.org/video/glossary.php

Autism Speaks provides a selection of videos illustrating behaviors commonly found in children with autism. These videos are available to everyone, but you must register with the organization before viewing.

www.challengingbehavior.org

This site provides a variety of information, from brief handouts to full articles, about supporting children with challenging behaviors.

www.nasponline.org/resources/handouts/Autism204_blue.pdf

Autism Spectrum Disorders: Primer for Parents and Educators by Lisa Ruble, PhD, and Trish Gallagher, MEd, presents a concise and readable explanation of autism spectrum disorders and effective educational interventions.

www.classroom-assistant.net

This site provides general resources for paraprofessional educators.

- *Assess implementation of CPRT regularly.* After your paraprofessionals can use all the components of CPRT correctly (yes, this will happen!), you still need to assess their implementation of CPRT on a regular basis. Regular assessment with feedback ensures that paraprofessionals will maintain their ability to use

| HANDOUT 17 | **Classroom Weekly Memo** | |

Dates: **10/19-10/23**

Classroom News:

Student half-day on F. Please be prepared for CPRT practice in the afternoon.

Jennifer's birthday on T; special snack time at 1:30.

Free workshop on autism at State College on Sat., Nov. 7 (we can register as a group now).

Student Updates:

Student	New Maintenance	New Acquisition	Preferences/Other
Julia	*Juice*	*Grapes, marker*	*Strawberry Shortcake; out on W, Th, F*
Brandon	*Kicking a ball, "I want" sentences*	*Kicking with direction, eat (food), play (toy)*	*Likes soccer ball*
Pramita	*Glitter, all colors*	*2-word phrases w/colors*	*Use colors with fingerpaints, ball drop*
David	*Tolerating peer nearby*	*Parallel play w/same toy/ activity w/peer*	*Dislikes puzzles; don't do puzzles with peer*
Liam	*Counting up to 20 (rote)*	*Counting w/correspondence up to 20*	*Will count anything!*

FIGURE 7.2. Completed Example of *Handout 17: Classroom Weekly Memo*. This form illustrates one method for keeping your classroom team updated on student goals and progress.

the components. Most people who learn something new will experience some loss of skill or drift over time. Your paraprofessionals may become so comfortable with CPRT that they make slight modifications to the intervention. Conversely, even paraprofessionals who have demonstrated mastery of all the components may still not feel confident using CPRT with different students in a variety of teaching situations. For these reasons, it is important to continue assessing your staff. We recommend making monthly assessments until a paraprofessional meets the fidelity criteria 3 months in a row, and then moving to quarterly assessments of fidelity.

Chapter Summary

Training paraprofessionals to use CPRT should enhance the overall learning experience of the students in your classroom. Although training paraprofessionals can be time-consuming, the resources and materials provided in this manual will facilitate the process of providing effective and ongoing training for your classroom staff.

CHAPTER 8

Parents as Partners
Sharing CPRT with Parents and Caregivers

CHAPTER OVERVIEW

Parents and other caregivers play a big role in their child's educational services, and it is important to communicate with parents about the teaching methods used in your classroom. This chapter provides information on how to share the basic structure and specific components of CPRT with the parents of students in your classroom. Handouts and tips to help parents implement CPRT in the home are also provided. Creating a partnership with parents will help students improve skills and increase responding both at home and at school.

The following sections are included:

Reasons for Involving Parents as Partners

Supporting Parents' Involvement
      Step 1: Provide Parents with the *CPRT in the Classroom* Handout
      Step 2: Provide Parents with the *CPRT at Home* Handout
      Step 3: Utilize the *CPRT Update* Form to Share Information

This chapter has a corresponding training lecture on the DVD accompanying this manual (*CPRT Session 5: Educating Paraprofessionals and Parents about CPRT*).

Parents and other caregivers play an important role in making educational decisions for their child. They are involved in the IEP process, their child's placement in a specific program or classroom, and the assessment and monitoring of their child's progress. As such, the parents of students in your classroom are interested in the teaching methods and strategies you are using to help their children make progress. In this chapter, we provide tools for sharing CPRT with parents and caregivers. The following information will help you tell parents about CPRT, as well as provide parents with the resources needed to implement this intervention at home.

Reasons for Involving Parents as Partners

At first, it may seem overwhelming to involve parents and caregivers with the interventions used in your classroom. Because there

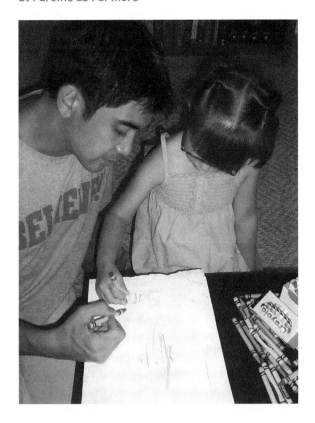

are already many pressures on you to provide a comprehensive education to each student, reaching out to parents in addition to managing your classroom from day to day may seem difficult. However, if you regularly share student goals and progress with parents and have a common approach to teaching, the growth you will see in student learning is well worth the extra effort!

Sharing CPRT with parents can lead to better progress over time and improve student responding, both at home and at school.

Research (see *Chapter 9*) shows that parents can learn to implement PRT reliably, leading to child gains in communication, play, and social skills. Also, parents find PRT more enjoyable to implement at home than other, more structured ABA-based programs because it can be used within the daily routines that they already complete

with their child, such as bath time, snack time, or play time. Parents have access to a wider variety of activities and settings with their child than those available at school, and they have unique knowledge about what motivates their child. They may also find that activities that used to be difficult—for example, getting a child dressed—become easier when CPRT strategies are used. Parents can use their child's preferences, such as wearing a favorite shirt or having certain toys in the bath, to increase their child's motivation while learning new skills. Though you will not be training and monitoring parents' use of CPRT the way you will with your paraprofessionals, parents can become valuable partners in addressing student goals outside the classroom. Utilize the unique opportunity presented by motivated parents by sharing CPRT with them.

Supporting Parents' Involvement

Just as effectively teaching students involves individualizing your approach to their unique needs and characteristics, sharing information with parents may require some individualization as well. The parents and caregivers of students in your classroom will come with a variety of levels of time, resources, energy, and availability. The process for sharing CPRT with parents suggested here allows you to tailor the amount of information you share. Although all parents can benefit from understanding the approach you are using in the classroom, not all parents may be equally able and/or motivated to implement CPRT at home. Some parents may already be feeling overwhelmed by the challenges of raising a child with autism. The best approach with these parents may be to share *Handout 18: CPRT in the Classroom* (provided in *Part IV*), as well as general notes about student progress and anecdotes from the school day, without making specific suggestions for addressing goals at home. There will be parents, however, who are eager to learn how they can interact with their child to promote new language, play, and social skills. These parents may be interested in reviewing the *CPRT Component Summary Sheets* (also available in *Part IV—Handouts 21–28*) and learning more about goal development.

> *Sharing CPRT with families can give you a common language to talk about the child's progress and the teaching methods you are using in the classroom.*

It is important to highlight to parents that CPRT is probably not a drastic change from the way they are currently interacting with their child. Instead, it is an approach to interaction in which they deliberately manage the antecedents (or cues) and consequences of their child's behavior to promote more positive responding in the future. It is likely to require slight modifications in how they respond to their child, but many of the components may be things they are already doing, such as providing direct rewards or reinforcing attempts. Taking the time to share CPRT with parents will empower them with tools to address their child's goals at home, and you are likely to see the benefits of this with your student in the classroom.

Take the following steps to share CPRT with your students' parents and caregivers, based on each family's need. Each step is discussed in more detail below. All handouts mentioned here are available in *Part IV* of the manual.

1. Provide parents with *Handout 18: CPRT in the Classroom*.

2. If parents are interested in learning more, provide them with *Handout 19: CPRT at Home*; *Handout 1: CPRT Components*;

and the *CPRT Component Summary Sheets* (*Handout 21–28*).

3. Utilize the *CPRT Update* forms (*Handouts 20A–20B*) to share information between home and the classroom.

> *Handouts 18, 19, 20A, and 20B in Part IV are available in both English and Spanish.*

Step 1: Provide Parents with *CPRT in the Classroom* Handout

Handout 18: CPRT in the Classroom is a one-page form that provides an overview of the ABC structure of CPRT and a list of the components. It also briefly discusses how data are collected during CPRT, as this is often a central question from concerned parents. This handout should be used as a first step to introduce parents to the approach you are using in your classroom. Because CPRT is naturalistic, someone who is not familiar with the approach may watch you interact with your students and not see the specific components you are using to promote learning. Many parents are more familiar with more structured ABA-based approaches and may be worried that their child is not receiving adequate intervention if they do not see a clear trial-based format.

> *Letting parents know exactly what you are doing may help them understand that their child is receiving high-quality, evidence-based intervention in the natural environment.*

Step 2: Provide Parents with *CPRT at Home* Handout

If parents ask for additional information about CPRT after learning that you are using the approach in your classroom, provide them with *Handout 19: CPRT at Home*. This more detailed handout condenses the information needed to understand the components of CPRT. The handout describes the eight CPRT components and the process of providing an opportunity to respond, observing the child's behavior, and responding with appropriate consequences. There is also a list of activity ideas for integrating CPRT into daily routines, and a brief list of resources for further information. You can also share the visual aid that lists all the components of CPRT for the parent to refer to at home (*Handout 1: CPRT Components*). If a parent requests more information on one or more specific components of CPRT, you can share the *CPRT Component Summary Sheets* (*Handouts 21–28*), the same way you might with your classroom staff.

Step 3: Utilize the *CPRT Update* Forms to Share Information

The two *CPRT Update* forms (*Handouts 20A and 20B*) allow two-way communication between you and your students' parents about student goals and progress. Research shows that parents are more likely to implement an intervention at home when they have a role in selecting goals. Informing parents about classroom activities can guide their choice of goals at home. Giving them a way to share with you the goals they are addressing at home can help motivate them to continue to use CPRT with their child.

The *CPRT Update* forms are designed to be passed between school and home on a regular basis. You and the parents will decide how often to share information with these forms. You can use *Handout 14: CPRT Student Profile* to fill out the information about student goals, as you will have probably already filled out that form

to share with your staff. The *CPRT Update* forms also allow you and the parents to share any activities or materials that may be particularly motivating to the student, as preferences are likely to change over time. In addition, *Handout 20A: CPRT Update— From Classroom to Home* contains a spot to highlight strategies that are particularly helpful in improving the student's responding in the classroom, such as gaining attention or allowing the child a choice of materials. Similarly, you can use *Handout 20B: CPRT Update—From Home to Classroom* to gather feedback from parents on what components they find most valuable at home.

It can often require creativity to incorporate student favorites into teaching specific skills, and surely two or three heads—both yours and the parents'—are better than one!

Chapter Summary

Your students' parents and other caregivers can become valuable partners when you share the approach you are using in your classroom and when they learn to implement CPRT at home. Materials and suggestions are provided here to individualize the information on CPRT you provide to parents, based on their level of motivation and availability. Sharing CPRT with parents/caregivers can give you a common language to talk about a child's progress, and it will empower parents with tools to address their child's goals at home. When you take the opportunity to involve parents, you are likely to see the benefits with your students in the classroom as well.

CHAPTER 9

Scientific Support for CPRT

CHAPTER OVERVIEW

CPRT is a direct adaptation of PRT, as noted in earlier chapters. PRT shares many features with other naturalistic behavioral techniques and has been used to address a wide range of behaviors. There is a large body of empirical research supporting the use of PRT to improve skills for children with autism. CPRT was developed to facilitate the incorporation of PRT strategies into today's classrooms.

The following sections are included:

History of CPRT

PRT Research
    Teaching Communication Using PRT
    Teaching Joint Attention Using PRT
    Teaching Play Skills Using PRT
    Teaching Peer Social Interaction Using PRT
    Using PRT to Improve Homework Skills

Adapting PRT for Use in the Classroom

As noted in earlier chapters, CPRT comes from a research-based program called PRT. PRT is a form of naturalistic behavioral intervention based on the principles of ABA, which is soundly supported in the scientific literature (National Research Council, 2001). ABA is the design, use, and evaluation of environmental modifications and interventions to produce socially significant improvement in human behavior (see *Chapter 2* for a detailed

description of ABA). ABA uses antecedent stimuli (things that happen before a behavior occurs, such as a teacher's asking a child the color of a crayon) and consequences (things that happen after a behavior occurs, such as giving the child the crayon after he names the color) to produce changes in behavior. ABA is based on the belief that we can shape an individual's behavior by altering environmental events that surround a behavior.

Treatments based on ABA represent a wide range of intervention strategies for children with autism, from highly structured programs conducted in one-on-one settings to naturalistic strategies that use a child's preferred activities to build skills.

History of CPRT

Naturalistic interventions have been developed to address some of the limitations associated with highly structured programs such as Discrete Trial Training (DTT; Lovaas, 1987). Thus the original PRT protocol was developed to help children respond to different cues, people, settings, and instructions; increase spontaneous responding; reduce dependency on prompts; and increase motivation—all while still relying on the principles of ABA.

Since their conception, naturalistic behavioral interventions have undergone a variety of changes and improvements. These changes have yielded several similar intervention techniques, including Incidental Teaching (Hart & Risley, 1968; McGee, Krantz, Mason, & McClannahan, 1983), the mand–model procedure (Rogers-Warren & Warren, 1980), time delay (Halle, Marshall, & Spradlin, 1979), Milieu Teaching (Alpert & Kaiser, 1992), and PRT (Koegel, O'Dell, & Koegel, 1987; Koegel, Schreibman, et al., 1988). Although specific techniques were developed in different laboratories, these approaches all share the following basic components (Delprato, 2001; Kaiser, Yoder, & Keetz, 1992):

- The learning environment is loosely structured.
- Teaching occurs within ongoing interactions between a child and an adult.

- The child initiates teaching episodes by indicating interest in an item or activity.
- Teaching materials are selected by the child and are varied often.
- The target behavior is explicitly prompted.
- A direct relationship exists between the child's response and the reinforcer.
- The child is reinforced for attempts to respond, not just for correct responses or successive approximations.

PRT was based on a series of empirical studies identifying important treatment elements that address "pivotal" areas of development affecting a wide range of functioning. According to Koegel and colleagues (1999), when these pivotal behaviors are enhanced, improvements in autonomy, self-learning, and generalization follow. PRT has been identified as an established intervention in a recent comprehensive review of treatment methods for use with children with autism conducted by the National Autism Center (2009; see also *www.nationalautismcenter.org/affiliates*).

To date, three pivotal areas have been identified: motivation, responsivity to multiple cues, and child self-initiations.

PRT Research

CPRT adapts the original PRT procedures for use in classroom settings. Because the systematic application of CPRT in classroom environments is relatively new, the bulk of the research on the use of the procedures has been conducted under the name PRT. Therefore, we use PRT to describe the research supporting the specific components of the program. In contrast to other naturalistic procedures that have focused mainly on communication, PRT has been used to teach a variety of skills, including symbolic play (Stahmer, 1995), sociodramatic play (Thorp, Stahmer, & Schreibman, 1995), peer social interaction (Pierce & Schreibman, 1995), self-initiations (Koegel, Carter, & Koegel, 2003), joint attention (Rocha, Schreibman, & Stahmer, 2007; Whalen & Schreibman, 2003), and homework completion (Koegel, Tran, Mossman, & Koegel, 2006). Independent reviews of the PRT research base recommend the program as an efficacious, evidence-based intervention for children with autism (Delprato, 2001; Humphries, 2003). Additionally, positive outcomes have been replicated by researchers not associated with the development of the original procedures (Jones, Carr, & Feeley, 2006; Kuhn, Bodkin, Devlin, & Doggett, 2008).

Teaching Communication Using PRT

A main focus of intervention for children with autism is communication. Communication affects many aspects of development; when students cannot communicate, it interferes with their ability to learn, delays their social development, and prevents them from achieving independence. Children with autism who do succeed in learning to communicate demonstrate lower levels of aberrant behaviors, such as self-stimulation, self-injury, tantrums, and aggression (Creedon, 1975). It is thus clear that the first goal of early intervention programs for children with autism should be to provide effective communication strategies.

Using PRT for students with autism (as described in *Chapter 3*) has led to better language improvements and fewer inappropriate and disruptive behaviors than has the use of traditional DTT methods (Koegel, Koegel, & Surratt, 1992). PRT has

been shown to be effective for improving speech imitation (Koegel, Camarata, Koegel, Ben-Tall, & Smith, 1998; Laski, Charlop, & Schreibman, 1988), labeling (Koegel, Camarata, Valdez-Menchaca, & Koegel, 1998), question asking (Koegel, Camarata, Valdez-Menchaca, & Koegel, 1998; Koegel et al., 2003), spontaneous speech (Laski et al., 1988), conversational communication (Koegel et al., 1998), and rapid acquisition of functional speech in previously nonverbal children (Sze, Koegel, Brookman, & Koegel, 2003). PRT has also been found to increase generalization (use of language skills in other settings and with other people) and maintenance (use of these skills over time) of communication changes in children with autism (Humphries, 2003; Schreibman, Kaneko, & Koegel, 1991). Spoken language has been the primary focus of much of the PRT research; therefore, it is clear that this technique is very effective at increasing spoken communication in children with autism (Humphries, 2003). Of course, as part of teaching communication, preacademic skills such as colors, numbers, letters, and shapes can be easily included as targets of the intervention (Koegel & Koegel, 2006).

Teaching Joint Attention Using PRT

In typical development, joint attention skills are considered to be pivotal behaviors leading to collateral changes in language (Bakeman & Adamson, 1984; Baron-Cohen, 1987; Bates, Benigni, Bretherton, Camaioni, & Volterra, 1979; Loveland & Landry, 1986). Children use joint attention with a social partner to communicate and learn about the environment. Joint attention is one of the core deficits in autism. Improving joint attention may improve other areas of development as well (Kasari et al., 2005). PRT has been used to directly teach joint attention skills (Pierce & Schreibman, 1995;

Whalen & Schreibman, 2003), and this has been associated with collateral changes in expressive language and social communication behaviors (Jones et al., 2006). For example, Whalen and Schreibman (2003) used PRT to teach joint attention to children with autism who learned to respond to showing, pointing, and gaze shifting of an adult; to coordinate gaze shifting (i.e., coordinated joint attention); and to point with the purpose of sharing, not requesting. These behaviors generalized to other settings, and naive observers using social validation measures noted positive changes.

Teaching Play Skills Using PRT

PRT has proven to be a naturalistic method that is structured enough to help children learn simple as well as more complex play skills, while still being flexible enough to allow children to play creatively. Research indicates that children with autism who are developmentally ready to learn symbolic and sociodramatic play skills can learn, via PRT, to engage in spontaneous, creative play with an adult at levels similar to those of language-age-matched peers (Humphries, 1998; Stahmer, 1995; Thorp et al., 1995). In one study, Stahmer (1995) used PRT to teach seven 4- to 6-year-old boys with autism who were developmentally ready to learn these skills to engage in symbolic play; the techniques described in the *Object Play Skills* section of *Chapter 5* were used. After 8 weeks of receiving PRT targeting symbolic play for 3 hours per week, the children significantly increased the number of spontaneous symbolic play behaviors they used, the complexity of their play, and the length and complexity of their interaction skills. The play skills taught using PRT showed generalization to new toys and adults, and these behavioral changes remained stable over time (Stahmer, 1995).

Teaching Peer Social Interaction Using PRT

Results from several PRT research projects indicate that it is an effective technique for teaching children with autism to respond to peers and to initiate interaction with others (Koegel et al., 1999; Kuhn et al., 2008; Pierce & Schreibman, 1997). For example, students with autism who participated in a PRT program had improved spontaneous social initiations and developed social circles of typically developing peers after treatment (Koegel et al., 1999). In one study, two 10-year-old boys with autism who had poor social skills and moderate developmental delays were taught to engage in social interactions using PRT. Prior to treatment, the children did not interact very much and never initiated such interactions with peers. After several weeks of training, however, both children maintained interactions with peers over 75% of the time, and started to initiate as well. Peer-implemented PRT led to changes in language and play that generalized to many settings, with different toys and new classmates. See the *Social Interaction Skills* section of *Chapter 5* for more specific methods for teaching social interaction.

Using PRT to Improve Homework Skills

PRT has been used to help children complete homework. Examples of PRT-based adaptations to homework include providing a choice of location to complete homework; providing a choice of order of completion, rather than choice of activity; interspersing simple problems (maintenance) with more difficult problems (acquisition); and rewarding attempts by rewarding the child for completing portions of a worksheet or attempting to complete a difficult problem (see the *Academic Skills* section of *Chapter 5*). When PRT procedures are used to help children do their homework, disruptive behaviors decrease, the children's positive affect increases, and homework performance improves (Koegel et al., 2006).

Adapting PRT for Use in the Classroom

Research examining how special educators usually teach young children with autism in the Southern California region indicated that over 70% of teachers surveyed reported using PRT or some variation of PRT in their programs (Stahmer, 2007). Twelve percent of the teachers using PRT, or seven total teachers, used it as the primary intervention in their program. Although PRT was their primary intervention, only two of the seven teachers reported that they used all aspects of the intervention. The remainder of these teachers indicated using parts of the intervention or using PRT in conjunction with other treatment methods. These finding suggested that collaboration with teachers was needed to make PRT user-friendly for the classroom. This was how CPRT was born.

We began by bringing together groups of teachers to ask them about the benefits and barriers associated with traditional PRT. Many teachers reported that PRT fit with their idea of "good teaching" and made sense to them. In addition, they reported that it helped children with autism generalize new skills to broader environments. They liked some of the specific steps of PRT, including keeping instructions and opportunities clear, simple, and relevant to the child; the use of maintenance tasks to keep child frustration low; the direct relationship between reinforcement and behavior; the ability to honor approximations and goal-directed attempts; and the use of explicit turn taking.

Preschool and elementary special education teachers found PRT to be an intuitive, effective teaching strategy for children with autism.

However, teachers also reported important barriers to the use of PRT in their classrooms. They found it difficult to take the skills they learned in one-on-one training and use them with groups of children (especially in settings such as circle time), in large classrooms, and without proper support. At times, they found it difficult to keep the multiple components straight; they also felt that having preliminary knowledge of ABA principles was an important prerequisite to understanding PRT. Moreover, teachers found data collection difficult and were unsure how to address specific IEP goals using PRT strategies. They felt that this was especially important, given that both parents and schools are data-driven and want programs to be determined by IEP goals. Teachers also asked for more information on how to train paraprofessionals in PRT. Furthermore, they felt that it was not always appropriate or possible for a child to choose an activity or for them to use direct reinforcement in the classroom. Finally, the use of multiple cues or conditional discriminations was an area of concern, especially for children who were minimally verbal. Based on this feedback, CPRT was developed as an adaptation of PRT to help teachers address IEP goals and teach in group settings using these strategies.

Although PRT has not been systematically studied in public school settings, there are some preliminary examples of classrooms using these procedures in combination with other strategies as part of their overall educational program. For example, the Children's Toddler School (now called Alexa's PLAYC, located at the Rady Children's Hospital, San Diego), an inclusive program for toddlers with autism, uses PRT with other interventions in daily programming. Teachers use PRT throughout the school day to encourage language, social, and preacademic skills (Stahmer & Ingersoll, 2004). The use of PRT is incorporated with the use of other strategies, such as DTT (Lovaas, 1987), PECS (Bondy & Frost, 1994), developmental/interactive techniques (Ingersoll & Dvortcsak, 2006), visual strategies (Schopler, Mesibov, & Hearsey, 1995), and sensory integration techniques (Baranek, 2002). In one study, although 50% of the children entered the Children's Toddler School program with no functional communication skills, 80% of children graduating from this program at age 3 had functional language. Moreover, approximately half of the children exited the program with conversational speech and cooperative symbolic play (Stahmer & Ingersoll, 2004).

Similarly, researchers in Oregon have been working with the Oregon State Department of Education to implement evidence-based practices in public school programs. A program was developed that included PRT along with other research-supported behavioral practices. Arick and colleagues (2003) reported outcome data for over 100 children with autism participating in the program, showing that the majority of children made significant progress in the areas of social interaction, expressive speech, and the use of language concepts. Children enrolled in the program gained, on average, more than 1 month of language age for every month of instruction. In addition, they displayed significant decreases in inappropriate/negative behaviors associated with autism. These findings are encouraging and support PRT as one part of an effective program for implementation in schools.

Chapter Summary

CPRT comes from a research-based program called PRT, a naturalistic behavioral intervention based on the principles of ABA. PRT was based on a series of empirical studies identifying important treatment elements that address "pivotal" areas of development affecting a wide range of functioning. PRT has been proven effective for teaching children with autism a wide variety of skills, including communication, joint attention, play, social interaction, and homework skills. Several independent reviews of the PRT research base recommend the program as an efficacious, evidence-based intervention for children with autism, and the positive child outcomes associated with it have been replicated by researchers not associated with PRT's development. CPRT adapts the original PRT procedures for use in classroom settings and is the product of close collaboration among researchers, teachers, and school administrators.

PART IV

Reproducible Handouts

CPRT Components

Cue

Student Attention
Be sure your student is paying attention before you provide a cue.

Clear and Appropriate Instruction
Provide clear and appropriate cues that are at, or just above, your student's developmental level.

Easy and Difficult Tasks (Maintenance/Acquisition)
Provide a mixture of easy and difficult tasks to increase motivation.

Shared Control (Student Choice/Turn Taking)
Share control by following your student's lead, providing choices of activities and materials, and taking turns with your student.

Multiple Cues (Broadening Attention)
Use multiple examples of materials and concepts to ensure broad understanding.

Present opportunities to respond that require your student to attend to multiple aspects of the learning materials.

Student Behavior or Response

Response

Direct Reinforcement
Provide reinforcement that is naturally or directly related to the activity or behavior.

Contingent Consequence (Immediate and Appropriate)
Present consequences immediately, based on the student's response.

Reinforcement of Attempts
Reward good trying to encourage your student to try again in the future.

Object Play Level Progression

When you begin working on your student's play skills, you will need to start at the level at which your student now interacts with objects, and move to more advanced levels one step at a time. The following list is designed to help you understand the progression of play skills and identify easy and difficult play skills for your student. Read the description of each type of play below, and circle either Yes, No, or Sometimes to indicate whether your student engages in this behavior. The Yes items will be maintenance tasks that you can utilize during play to keep student motivation high. The Sometimes items will be acquisition tasks, and you will help your student learn to use these play skills more consistently. You should model play that is one level above your student's current abilities (Yes and Sometimes items) as you take turns during play with your student. Your student may be learning several similar levels of play at one time, but you should generally be sure that your student has mastered each of the previous levels of play before moving on to more advanced skills.

Sensory Exploration			
Uses senses to explore objects Some students begin to play by using their senses. They may put objects in their mouths, sniff objects, visually expect objects, etc. Often at this stage students will perform the same action with all objects or toys, such as banging, shaking, or spinning. Does your student *currently* use this form of play? Circle *one:*	Yes	No	Sometimes
Repetitive sensory exploration During this stage of play, some students will engage in one form of sensory play ritualistically or repetitively for extended periods of time. Some students will engage in this behavior so much that they do not play any other way very often. Does your student *currently* use this form of play? Circle *one:*	Yes	No	Sometimes
Object exploration Some students explore object by looking for differences in shape, color, texture, etc. During this stage, they may be turning, pulling, poking, and tearing objects. Students at this stage use one object at a time and change items often. They are not yet putting objects together or understanding cause-and-effect play. Does your student *currently* use this form of play? Circle *one:*	Yes	No	Sometimes
Early Relational Play			
Cause-and-effect play Students at this stage often begin to combine objects, such as putting objects in a container, pushing buttons, turning handles, opening and shutting, etc. Students at this stage may begin to throw in play (not just to get rid of an object). Students may put some actions together and begin to have some interest in toys such as busy boxes, shape sorters, etc. Does your student *currently* use this form of play? Circle *one:*	Yes	No	Sometimes
Relational play Students at this stage begin to use toys more functionally—for example, throwing a ball, pushing a toy car, blowing a noisemaker, placing pegs in a hole, etc. During this stage, play becomes more purposeful. Does your student *currently* use this form of play? Circle *one:*	Yes	No	Sometimes
Symbolic or Pretend Play			
Early pretend play—directed toward self Students begin pretending by doing familiar actions toward themselves. Students may pretend to eat, drink, sleep, comb hair, and talk on the phone as their earliest form of pretend. Students at this stage use realistic objects and may add sound effects (such as lip smacking for eating). Does your student *currently* use this form of play? Circle *one:*	Yes	No	Sometimes

(cont.)

Symbolic or Pretend Play *(cont.)*			
Early pretend play—directed toward others Students then begin to pretend toward other people. Students at this stage may pretend to feed you or a sibling, and perhaps a doll. Feeding and grooming are often seen first. Your student may begin to link actions such as putting a doll in a car at this stage. Does your student *currently* use this form of play? Circle *one:*	Yes	No	Sometimes
Linking early pretend actions Once students have practiced these early pretend actions, they may begin to perform the same action on multiple play partners—for example, feed self, feed mom, feed dad, feed doll; drink from several cups; etc. Does your student *currently* use this form of play? Circle *one:*	Yes	No	Sometimes
Early symbolic object play After using realistic objects in play, students begin to use substitute objects, such as pretending that a block is a cookie or a rope is a hose. Substitute objects often look similar to the real object. Students may also pretend to pour juice or that a toy stove is hot in this stage. Does your student *currently* use this form of play? Circle *one:*	Yes	No	Sometimes
Symbolic sounds and gestures Students may use sound effects such as "vroom" when racing a car or "choo-choo" for a train. They may say "ouch" when a doll falls down or give a voice to a doll. Does your student *currently* use this form of play? Circle *one:*	Yes	No	Sometimes
Linking symbolic actions Once students use a variety of pretend play actions, they begin to link these actions. They might put gas in a car and then drive the car, or brush a doll's teeth and put the doll to bed. Dolls are still passive partners. Does your student *currently* use this form of play? Circle *one:*	Yes	No	Sometimes
Doll as active agent Next, students begin to make the dolls active agents in play. A doll is made to wash itself, walk, or hold a spoon. Does your student *currently* use this form of play? Circle *one:*	Yes	No	Sometimes
Advanced substitute object use Next, we begin to expect students to search for a missing or substitute object to use in pretend play. They may look for an item to be pretend food or a pretend car; they may pretend to wash a car without any water. Substitute objects may not look anything like the real object. Does your student *currently* use this form of play? Circle *one:*	Yes	No	Sometimes
Telling stories with toys As students become good at symbolic play, they begin to act out more complex stories with toys. For example, they may put gas in a car, drive the car, crash the car, fix the car, etc., all as part of one play sequence. They may feed a doll with a bottle, pat it on the back and put it to bed or put pretend toothpaste on a toothbrush, put the cap on the tube, and brush the doll's teeth. Dolls may take multiple roles. Does your student *currently* use this form of play? Circle *one:*	Yes	No	Sometimes

(cont.)

Sociodramatic Play			
Acting things out			
At the most complex level, students will begin to assign one or multiple roles to themselves or other friends, starting with familiar fantasy themes and moving to fantasy characters and stories they create. This play may be supported by props or simply by language and gesture. This type of play can be very elaborate and can be difficult for students with autism. Does your student *currently* use this form of play? Circle *one*:	Yes	No	Sometimes
Games with Rules			
Simple games			
Learning games occurs along with object play. Students begin to learn to take turns, and follow directions in the context of games. Chase type games, and simple games of catch are examples of the first forms of game play students typically learn. Does your student *currently* use this form of play? Circle *one*:	Yes	No	Sometimes
Manipulative games			
There are some simple games with few rules or steps that also have a manipulative component, and these can be excellent first games—for example, a game such as Don't Break the Ice. Does your student *currently* use this form of play? Circle *one*:	Yes	No	Sometimes
Board games			
As students begin to understand problem solving and rules, they can move to more complicated board games that include academic skills, turn taking, and winning–losing. Does your student *currently* use this form of play? Circle *one*:	Yes	No	Sometimes
Organized sports/playground games			
Students can play organized large motor games at a variety of levels, from playing handball to an organized game of baseball. Tasks should be broken down into small steps to help determine how much assistance a student will need to participate in this type of game. Does your student *currently* use this form of play? Circle *one*:	Yes	No	Sometimes
Additional Play Behaviors			

Stereotyped play	If Yes, model new ways to play with that toy or build on your student's favorite action to vary it slightly.		
Some students have advanced play skills, but play only with a particular toy or complete the same action or sequence with every toy they encounter. Does your student *currently* use this form of play? Circle *one*:	Yes	No	Sometimes

Duration of play	If Yes, slowly increase the amount of time required with a toy before moving forward.		
Some students have a difficult time staying with one toy for extended period of time and may move quickly between available toys. Does your student move frequently (more than once per minute) between toys and activities? Circle *one*:	Yes	No	Sometimes

Facilitated play	If Yes, work on spontaneous play and initiation of play activities before moving forward with higher levels of prompted play.		
Some students play at higher levels only when a teacher or other adult is helping them play, and do not demonstrate these play skills independently. For the highest levels of play you circled above, does your student only engage in these with your help? Circle *one*:	Yes	No	Sometimes

156

Gathering Information

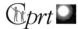

Student: _____

We need your help! We know that your experience with _____
will be very helpful as we welcome him/her into our classroom. Please take a few minutes to tell us what he/
she likes. Be specific. We will use this information to keep him/her motivated to learn and interested in classroom
activities. Thank you for your help!

Completed by: _____   Relationship to student: _____

What does he/she enjoy?

What	How	How much (3 = high)	When
Example: Playing on computer (alphabet game)	*Likes to match capital to lower-case letters (alone only; has trouble sharing)*	1 ② 3	*Good as a transition back to classroom after lunch or morning recess*
Example: Graham crackers	*Whole or half crackers; rejects crackers that are broken unevenly*	1 2 ③	*Any time*
		1 2 3	
		1 2 3	
		1 2 3	
		1 2 3	
		1 2 3	
		1 2 3	
		1 2 3	

Any other tips or comments? _____
_____
_____

CPRT Time-Based Preference Assessment

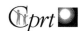

Student: _____ Date: _____

Choose a set of 10 items available in your classroom that you think the student might like. List each item (toy, food item, etc.) below.

Items	Number of times chosen	Rank		Ranked items	Preference level
1.					High
2.					High
3.					High
4.					Medium
5.					Medium
6.					Medium
7.					Low
8.					Low
9.					Low
10.					Low

Gather all the items, and make them all easily accessible to the student. Prior to the assessment, allow the student to try each of the items. Set a timer to sound every 10 seconds. When the timer goes off, indicate which item(s) the student is playing with or consuming by circling the number that corresponds with the item listed above. Replenish any food items during the assessment if necessary.

Interval	Item engaged with (circle)										Interval	Item engaged with (circle)									
1	1	2	3	4	5	6	7	8	9	10	16	1	2	3	4	5	6	7	8	9	10
2	1	2	3	4	5	6	7	8	9	10	17	1	2	3	4	5	6	7	8	9	10
3	1	2	3	4	5	6	7	8	9	10	18	1	2	3	4	5	6	7	8	9	10
4	1	2	3	4	5	6	7	8	9	10	19	1	2	3	4	5	6	7	8	9	10
5	1	2	3	4	5	6	7	8	9	10	20	1	2	3	4	5	6	7	8	9	10
6	1	2	3	4	5	6	7	8	9	10	21	1	2	3	4	5	6	7	8	9	10
7	1	2	3	4	5	6	7	8	9	10	22	1	2	3	4	5	6	7	8	9	10
8	1	2	3	4	5	6	7	8	9	10	23	1	2	3	4	5	6	7	8	9	10
9	1	2	3	4	5	6	7	8	9	10	24	1	2	3	4	5	6	7	8	9	10
10	1	2	3	4	5	6	7	8	9	10	25	1	2	3	4	5	6	7	8	9	10
11	1	2	3	4	5	6	7	8	9	10	26	1	2	3	4	5	6	7	8	9	10
12	1	2	3	4	5	6	7	8	9	10	27	1	2	3	4	5	6	7	8	9	10
13	1	2	3	4	5	6	7	8	9	10	28	1	2	3	4	5	6	7	8	9	10
14	1	2	3	4	5	6	7	8	9	10	29	1	2	3	4	5	6	7	8	9	10
15	1	2	3	4	5	6	7	8	9	10	30	1	2	3	4	5	6	7	8	9	10

Count the number of time points at which the student was engaged with each item. Then rank the items from the most often selected to the least often. Highly preferred items are the three items the student selected most often, moderately preferred items are the three items selected the next most often, and so forth (see scale on right).

Other notes: _____

_____

_____

_____

CPRT Paired-Choice Preference Assessment

Student: _____ Date: _____

Choose a set of six items available in your classroom that you think the student might like. List each item (toy, food item, etc.) below. Gather all items so they are easily accessible throughout the assessment.

Stimulus	Percent chosen			Preference level		
1.	/10 =		%	High	Medium	Low
2.	/10 =		%	High	Medium	Low
3.	/10 =		%	High	Medium	Low
4.	/10 =		%	High	Medium	Low
5.	/10 =		%	High	Medium	Low
6.	/10 =		%	High	Medium	Low

On each trial, select the two items associated with the item numbers listed below. Place both items in front of the student. Record each item the student selects from the pair, and allow the student to interact briefly with the item. If the student does not select either item, pause the assessment and present each item one at a time, prompting the student to interact with it if necessary. Then re-present the trial. If the student does not select either item on the second presentation of the pair, move on. Block any attempts to access both items by removing the items and re-presenting the pair later in the assessment.

Trial	Left	Right	Item selected
1	1	2	
2	3	4	
3	5	6	
4	2	3	
5	4	5	
6	1	3	
7	2	4	
8	3	5	
9	4	6	
10	1	4	
11	3	6	
12	2	5	
13	6	1	
14	1	5	
15	2	6	

Trial	Left	Right	Item selected
16	4	1	
17	6	3	
18	5	2	
19	1	6	
20	5	1	
21	6	2	
22	2	1	
23	4	3	
24	6	5	
25	3	2	
26	5	4	
27	3	1	
28	4	2	
29	5	3	
30	6	4	

Calculate the percent of trials in which the student selected each item. Each item was presented 10 times. The percentage of trials in which an item was selected can be determined by dividing the number of times the item was selected by 10. Highly preferred items are those selected in 80% or more of the trials. Moderately preferred items are those selected in 40–70%. Low-preference items are selected in less than 40% of the trials.

Other notes: _____
_____
_____

CPRT Planning and Progress

Student: _____

This form is designed to facilitate planning and progress tracking related to IEP goals and curriculum areas. Enter goals that can be optimally targeted using CPRT on the grid below. For each goal, think of 1–3 classroom settings or activities in which this goal can be addressed with CPRT. List the activity ideas and the date of goal introduction in the spaces provided. **Each month**, mark the date of the Progress Assessment (PA) and review the relevant *CPRT Goal Summary* sheets for the specified goals. If the student has met the goal, circle A for Achieved and draw a line through the remaining PA columns. If the student is making progress but has not yet met the mastery criteria for a particular goal, circle O for Ongoing and continue addressing the goal through CPRT. If a student is not making progress on a goal despite correct and consistent implementation of CPRT, circle D for Discontinue and consider alternative strategies to reach this goal. Transfer Ongoing goals to a new *CPRT Planning and Progress* sheet after three Progress Assessments.

KEY

A: Achieved; student has met mastery criteria for this goal.

O: Ongoing; student is making progress and the goal will continue to be addressed through CPRT

D: Discontinue; student is making no progress on this goal; consider alternative strategies.

IEP or Curriculum Area Goal	Activities/Settings	Date Introduced	PA 1 Date: _____	PA 2 Date: _____	PA 3 Date: _____
			A O D	A O D	A O D
			A O D	A O D	A O D
			A O D	A O D	A O D
			A O D	A O D	A O D
			A O D	A O D	A O D
			A O D	A O D	A O D
			A O D	A O D	A O D

CPRT Goal Summary

Student: _____

This form is designed to track student progress on goals being addressed with CPRT. Write the curriculum area or IEP goal in the space provided, and enter the first step to reaching the goal in the grid below. Enter the date that this benchmark or step was introduced. On each data collection day, transfer data from one of the *CPRT Data Records* to this sheet. Depending on which *CPRT Data Record* was used, enter the plus/check/minus rating and support level typically required to elicit the target skill (from *CPRT Data Record: Unstructured* or *CPRT Data Record: Semistructured*) or the exact measurement of goal progress (from *CPRT Data Record: Structured*). After four data collection days (a Period), use the measurements listed to determine if the step is Achieved (A) or Ongoing (O), and circle the appropriate option. This will allow you to assess progress on the goal over time and to determine necessary next steps for your student and teaching staff.

Goal: _____

Benchmark/Step or Procedure Changes		Period 1						Period 2						Period 3						Period 4					
		1	2	3	4	A	O	1	2	3	4	A	O	1	2	3	4	A	O	1	2	3	4	A	O
	Date					A	O					A	O					A	O					A	O
	Date					A	O					A	O					A	O					A	O
	Date					A	O					A	O					A	O					A	O
	Date					A	O					A	O					A	O					A	O
	Date					A	O					A	O					A	O					A	O

CPRT Data Record: Unstructured

Student: _____   Date: _____

To use this data record, complete one row each time you use CPRT with your student. This method does not require data collection during the interaction with the student. Complete the row at the end of the interaction, and note the length of the interaction in the appropriate column. Use the key below to indicate the student's general level of responding for both acquisition and maintenance skills, prompts used, and level of motivation and compliance.

KEY:

+ = Responds independently to all or almost all (at least 80%) opportunities

✓ = Responds independently to most opportunities (50%), but requires support for some opportunities

– = Requires support to respond to all or almost all opportunities

Prompt Level:
F: Full or **P:** Partial

Prompt Type:
Ph: Physical, **V:** Verbal, **Vs:** Visual, **G:** Gestural

Motivation/Compliance:
1—Optimal motivation, minimal negative behaviors
2—High motivation, few negative behaviors
3—Good motivation, some negative behaviors
4—Poor motivation, moderate negative behaviors
5—Minimal motivation, many negative behaviors

Date	Teacher	Activity/materials + length of time	Goal/curriculum area	Acquisition skills	+ ✓ –	Sample best acquisition skill response (include prompt level, if any)	Most frequent prompt level (if any)	Maintenance skills	+ ✓ –	Motivation
										1 2 3 4 5
										1 2 3 4 5
										1 2 3 4 5
										1 2 3 4 5

(cont.)

CPRT Data Record: Unstructured *(page 2 of 2)*

Date	Teacher	Activity/materials + length of time	Goal/curriculum area	Acquisition skills	+ ✓ −	Sample best acquisition skill response (include prompt level, if any)	Most frequent prompt level (if any)	Maintenance skills	+ ✓ −	Motivation
										1 2 3 4 5
										1 2 3 4 5
										1 2 3 4 5
										1 2 3 4 5
										1 2 3 4 5
										1 2 3 4 5
										1 2 3 4 5

CPRT Data Record: Semistructured

Student: _____ Date: _____

To use this data record, record data during natural pauses in the activity every 3–5 minutes. **Before you begin CPRT:** Enter the goals to be addressed with CPRT in the spaces provided, and define maintenance and acquisition skills or targets for the student. **During the activity:** After each interval, record the materials and the type of support used *most often* to elicit the *acquisition skills*. Record sample student responses for the acquisition skills at the support level indicated. At each interval, rate the student's performance of maintenance skills for that goal, based on the key below.

Support Level:
F: Full or **P:** Partial

Support Type:
Ph: Physical, **V:** Verbal,
Vs: Visual, **G:** Gestural,
I: Independent (no support)

KEY:
+ = Responds independently to all or almost all (at least 80%) opportunities

✓ = Responds independently to most opportunities (50%), but requires support for some opportunities

− = Requires support to respond to all or almost all opportunities

Goal/Curriculum Area: _____

Maintenance Skill: _____ **Acquisition Skill:** _____

Initials	Material/Activity	Support		Acq. +/✓/−	Sample Student Response/Notes	Maint. +/✓/−
		F / P	Ph V Vs G I			
		F / P	Ph V Vs G I			
		F / P	Ph V Vs G I			
		F / P	Ph V Vs G I			
SUMMARY	Most frequent level of response:			Most frequent support level:		

Goal/Curriculum Area: _____

Maintenance Skill: _____ **Acquisition Skill:** _____

Initials	Material/Activity	Support		Acq. +/✓/−	Sample Student Response/Notes	Maint. +/✓/−
		F / P	Ph V Vs G I			
		F / P	Ph V Vs G I			
		F / P	Ph V Vs G I			
		F / P	Ph V Vs G I			
SUMMARY	Most frequent level of response:			Most frequent support level:		

(cont.)

Goal/Curriculum Area: _____

Maintenance Skill: _____ Acquisition Skill: _____

Initials	Material/Activity	Support		Acq. +/✓/–	Sample Student Response/Notes	Maint. +/✓/–
		F / P	Ph V Vs G I			
		F / P	Ph V Vs G I			
		F / P	Ph V Vs G I			
		F / P	Ph V Vs G I			
SUMMARY	Most frequent level of response:			Most frequent support level:		

Goal/Curriculum Area: _____

Maintenance Skill: _____ Acquisition Skill: _____

Initials	Material/Activity	Support		Acq. +/✓/–	Sample Student Response/Notes	Maint. +/✓/–
		F / P	Ph V Vs G I			
		F / P	Ph V Vs G I			
		F / P	Ph V Vs G I			
		F / P	Ph V Vs G I			
SUMMARY	Most frequent level of response:			Most frequent support level:		

Goal/Curriculum Area: _____

Maintenance Skill: _____ Acquisition Skill: _____

Initials	Material/Activity	Support		Acq. +/✓/–	Sample Student Response/Notes	Maint. +/✓/–
		F / P	Ph V Vs G I			
		F / P	Ph V Vs G I			
		F / P	Ph V Vs G I			
		F / P	Ph V Vs G I			
SUMMARY	Most frequent level of response:			Most frequent support level:		

CPRT Data Record: Structured

Student: _____ Date: _____

To use this data record, take data on each individual trial in which you present an opportunity to respond to your student. Enter goals to be addressed with CPRT in the spaces provided, and define maintenance and acquisition skills for each goal. In each trial column, indicate whether you targeted a maintenance or acquisition skill, the child's response, and the support level used (if any; you may also just make a mark in the support box if you are not gathering support-type information). At the end of the session, calculate the total number or percent of acquisition trials in which the child responded correctly and independently (number of acquisition trials correct and independent/total number of acquisition trials), depending on what is being measured. Enter this information at the top of each box. Use the Comments section to indicate any important information about that particular goal, such as difficulty with maintenance skills or helpful materials. Use the General Notes section to indicate overall impressions from the session, including student affect, motivation level, and inappropriate behaviors.

Because you will be using CPRT in the context of play and other semistructured activities, intensive trial-by-trial data collection can inhibit the natural flow of interaction between you and your student. To resolve this issue, try completing three to four trials, then allowing the child extended access to the activity materials while you record the data.

Response:
+: Correct response
Att: Attempt toward correct response
–: Incorrect response
NR: No response

Support Level:
F: Full or **P:** Partial

Support Type:
Ph: Physical, **V:** Verbal, **Vs:** Visual, **G:** Gestural

Teacher:		Goal:											Acquisition Trials Correct (% or #):						
Acquisition Skill:																			
Maintenance Skill:																			
Trial	1	2	3	4	5	6	7	8	9	10	11	12	13	14	15	16	17	18	19	20
Target	M A	M A	M A	M A	M A	M A	M A	M A	M A	M A	M A	M A	M A	M A	M A	M A	M A	M A	M A	M A
Response	+ Att – NR	+ Att – NR	+ Att – NR	+ Att – NR	+ Att – NR	+ Att – NR	+ Att – NR	+ Att – NR	+ Att – NR	+ Att – NR	+ Att – NR	+ Att – NR	+ Att – NR	+ Att – NR	+ Att – NR	+ Att – NR	+ Att – NR	+ Att – NR	+ Att – NR	+ Att – NR
Prompt																				
Comments:																				

Teacher:		Goal:											Acquisition Trials Correct (% or #):						
Acquisition Skill:																			
Maintenance Skill:																			
Trial	1	2	3	4	5	6	7	8	9	10	11	12	13	14	15	16	17	18	19	20
Target	M A	M A	M A	M A	M A	M A	M A	M A	M A	M A	M A	M A	M A	M A	M A	M A	M A	M A	M A	M A
Response	+ Att – NR	+ Att – NR	+ Att – NR	+ Att – NR	+ Att – NR	+ Att – NR	+ Att – NR	+ Att – NR	+ Att – NR	+ Att – NR	+ Att – NR	+ Att – NR	+ Att – NR	+ Att – NR	+ Att – NR	+ Att – NR	+ Att – NR	+ Att – NR	+ Att – NR	+ Att – NR
Prompt																				
Comments:																				

(cont.)

Teacher:		Goal:										Acquisition Trials Correct (% or #):								
Acquisition Skill:																				
Maintenance Skill:																				
Trial	1	2	3	4	5	6	7	8	9	10	11	12	13	14	15	16	17	18	19	20
Target	M A	M A	M A	M A	M A	M A	M A	M A	M A	M A	M A	M A	M A	M A	M A	M A	M A	M A	M A	M A
Response	+ Att − NR	+ Att − NR	+ Att − NR	+ Att − NR	+ Att − NR	+ Att − NR	+ Att − NR	+ Att − NR	+ Att − NR	+ Att − NR	+ Att − NR	+ Att − NR	+ Att − NR	+ Att − NR	+ Att − NR	+ Att − NR	+ Att − NR	+ Att − NR	+ Att − NR	+ Att − NR
Prompt																				
Comments:																				

Teacher:		Goal:										Acquisition Trials Correct (% or #):								
Acquisition Skill:																				
Maintenance Skill:																				
Trial	1	2	3	4	5	6	7	8	9	10	11	12	13	14	15	16	17	18	19	20
Target	M A	M A	M A	M A	M A	M A	M A	M A	M A	M A	M A	M A	M A	M A	M A	M A	M A	M A	M A	M A
Response	+ Att − NR	+ Att − NR	+ Att − NR	+ Att − NR	+ Att − NR	+ Att − NR	+ Att − NR	+ Att − NR	+ Att − NR	+ Att − NR	+ Att − NR	+ Att − NR	+ Att − NR	+ Att − NR	+ Att − NR	+ Att − NR	+ Att − NR	+ Att − NR	+ Att − NR	+ Att − NR
Prompt																				
Comments:																				

Teacher:		Goal:										Acquisition Trials Correct (% or #):								
Acquisition Skill:																				
Maintenance Skill:																				
Trial	1	2	3	4	5	6	7	8	9	10	11	12	13	14	15	16	17	18	19	20
Target	M A	M A	M A	M A	M A	M A	M A	M A	M A	M A	M A	M A	M A	M A	M A	M A	M A	M A	M A	M A
Response	+ Att − NR	+ Att − NR	+ Att − NR	+ Att − NR	+ Att − NR	+ Att − NR	+ Att − NR	+ Att − NR	+ Att − NR	+ Att − NR	+ Att − NR	+ Att − NR	+ Att − NR	+ Att − NR	+ Att − NR	+ Att − NR	+ Att − NR	+ Att − NR	+ Att − NR	+ Att − NR
Prompt																				
Comments:																				

General Notes:

CPRT Group Data Record: Tally

Activity: _____ Teacher: _____ Date: _____

This sheet allows you to keep data during group instruction. Though not all students have identical goals, grouping those with similar goals will help you use this form.

Before the activity begins: Write several goals relevant to the activity across the top of the grid below, and list the participating students on the left. Make a note of the current acquisition skill for each student in each column. **During the activity:** Record data by tallying the number of times each student demonstrates the skill independently (Ind) and with prompting (Pmt). Taking data while teaching a group of students is a learned skill, but with practice it is possible to conduct group instruction while tracking student responses. To start, you may want to record data on one student for an interval of time and then switch to a second student, and so forth, or select one or two students to track each day, so that data collection remains manageable.

Student	Goal/Behavior:	Goal/Behavior:	Goal/Behavior:	Motivation
	Skill: Ind: Pmt: Miss Opp:	Skill: Ind: Pmt: Miss Opp:	Skill: Ind: Pmt: Miss Opp:	1 2 3 4 5
	Skill: Ind: Pmt: Miss Opp:	Skill: Ind: Pmt: Miss Opp:	Skill: Ind: Pmt: Miss Opp:	1 2 3 4 5
	Skill: Ind: Pmt: Miss Opp:	Skill: Ind: Pmt: Miss Opp:	Skill: Ind: Pmt: Miss Opp:	1 2 3 4 5
	Skill: Ind: Pmt: Miss Opp:	Skill: Ind: Pmt: Miss Opp:	Skill: Ind: Pmt: Miss Opp:	1 2 3 4 5
	Skill: Ind: Pmt: Miss Opp:	Skill: Ind: Pmt: Miss Opp:	Skill: Ind: Pmt: Miss Opp:	1 2 3 4 5

From *Classroom Pivotal Response Teaching for Children with Autism* by Aubyn C. Stahmer, Jessica Suhrheinrich, Sarah Reed, Laura Schreibman, and Cynthia Bolduc. Copyright 2011 by The Guilford Press. Permission to photocopy this handout is granted to purchasers of this book for personal use only (see copyright page for details).

CPRT Group Data Record: Rating

Activity: _____   Teacher: _____   Date: _____

This sheet allows you to keep data during group instruction. Though not all students have identical goals, grouping those with similar goals will help you use this form.

Before the activity begins: Write several goals relevant to the activity across the top of the grid below, and list the participating students on the left. Make a note of the current acquisition skill for each student in each column. **During the activity:** Record data by rating each student's performance of the acquisition skill from 1 to 5 at three points during the activity. Use the rating scale below. It may be easiest to set a timer for one-third the planned length of the activity and record data when the timer sounds. Alternatively, it may be helpful to rate one student in all areas every few minutes, so that data collection remains manageable. At the end, rate each student's motivation from 1 to 5. To start, you may want to record data on one student for an interval of time and then switch to a second student, and so forth, or select one or two students to track each day, so that data collection remains manageable.

1: No response/maximal prompting required at all opportunities

2: Maximal prompting required at most opportunities; no independent responses

3: Some prompting required at most opportunities; sporadic independent responses

4: Some independent responses (at least 50%); some prompted responses

5: Primarily independent responses (more than 75% of responses independent)

Student	Goal				Goal				Goal				Goal				Motivation
	Skill: Rating: 1 2 3 4 5 1 2 3 4 5 1 2 3 4 5				Skill: Rating: 1 2 3 4 5 1 2 3 4 5 1 2 3 4 5				Skill: Rating: 1 2 3 4 5 1 2 3 4 5 1 2 3 4 5				Skill: Rating: 1 2 3 4 5 1 2 3 4 5 1 2 3 4 5				1 2 3 4 5
	Skill: Rating: 1 2 3 4 5 1 2 3 4 5 1 2 3 4 5				Skill: Rating: 1 2 3 4 5 1 2 3 4 5 1 2 3 4 5				Skill: Rating: 1 2 3 4 5 1 2 3 4 5 1 2 3 4 5				Skill: Rating: 1 2 3 4 5 1 2 3 4 5 1 2 3 4 5				1 2 3 4 5
	Skill: Rating: 1 2 3 4 5 1 2 3 4 5 1 2 3 4 5				Skill: Rating: 1 2 3 4 5 1 2 3 4 5 1 2 3 4 5				Skill: Rating: 1 2 3 4 5 1 2 3 4 5 1 2 3 4 5				Skill: Rating: 1 2 3 4 5 1 2 3 4 5 1 2 3 4 5				1 2 3 4 5
	Skill: Rating: 1 2 3 4 5 1 2 3 4 5 1 2 3 4 5				Skill: Rating: 1 2 3 4 5 1 2 3 4 5 1 2 3 4 5				Skill: Rating: 1 2 3 4 5 1 2 3 4 5 1 2 3 4 5				Skill: Rating: 1 2 3 4 5 1 2 3 4 5 1 2 3 4 5				1 2 3 4 5

CPRT Generalization Probe

Student: _____

Goal Domain: _____ Benchmark: _____

To ensure that a skill target is functional for your student, you must know if he/she can use this skill in a variety of circumstances. Identify three different materials, settings, and teachers for the purpose of probing the skill listed above. The materials you choose should be highly preferred by the student.

Materials/Activity: 1.
                    2.
                    3.

Setting: 1.
             2.
             3.

Partner: 1.
             2.
             3.

Indicate the date and the circumstances in which you will probe the skill. Circle the number that corresponds with the specific materials, setting, or teacher listed above. Circle the student's response to the probed skill target as Correct (C), Incorrect (I), or No Response (NR).

Date	Materials			Setting			Teacher			Student Response		
	1	2	3	1	2	3	1	2	3	C	I	NR
	1	2	3	1	2	3	1	2	3	C	I	NR
	1	2	3	1	2	3	1	2	3	C	I	NR
	1	2	3	1	2	3	1	2	3	C	I	NR
	1	2	3	1	2	3	1	2	3	C	I	NR
	1	2	3	1	2	3	1	2	3	C	I	NR
	1	2	3	1	2	3	1	2	3	C	I	NR
	1	2	3	1	2	3	1	2	3	C	I	NR
	1	2	3	1	2	3	1	2	3	C	I	NR
	1	2	3	1	2	3	1	2	3	C	I	NR
	1	2	3	1	2	3	1	2	3	C	I	NR
	1	2	3	1	2	3	1	2	3	C	I	NR
	1	2	3	1	2	3	1	2	3	C	I	NR
	1	2	3	1	2	3	1	2	3	C	I	NR
Total												

Summary: _____

_____

_____

CPRT Student Profile

Student: _____

This form is designed to facilitate communication about a student's preferences and current ability level. Update progress and preferences regularly (weekly is suggested), and share this document with your team. Use the *CPRT Data Record* forms to gather information to complete this profile.

Benchmark/Goal:			
Date	**Acquisition**	**Maintenance**	**Preferences**

Benchmark/Goal:			

(cont.)

Benchmark/Goal:			
Date	Acquisition	Maintenance	Preferences

Benchmark/Goal:			

Notes:

CPRT Assessment

Teacher: _____ Observer: _____ Date: _____

Activity: _____

Score each component based on your observation of the teacher–student interaction. After scoring each component, provide a summary score for the intervention technique that best captures how the teacher performed on the components. To achieve fidelity, the teacher must receive a score of 4 or 5 on each of the technique summary scores. If the child is not developmentally ready, or does not have difficulty with discrimination, mark N/A for multiple cues.

List the maintenance (easy) tasks and acquisition (difficult) tasks for this student:

Low Fidelity 1	2	3	4	High Fidelity 5
Teacher does not implement throughout session.	Teacher implements occasionally, but misses majority of opportunities.	Teacher implements up to half of the time, but misses many opportunities.	Teacher implements a majority of the time, but misses some opportunities.	Teacher implements throughout the session.

Intervention Technique	Fidelity	Notes
Teacher maximizes student motivation		
Follows student's lead, provides choices of activities and materials	1 2 3 4 5	
Takes turns with the student and/or facilitates turns among students	1 2 3 4 5	
Provides a mixture of easy and difficult tasks to increase motivation (maintenance/acquisition)	1 2 3 4 5	
Summary	*1 2 3 4 5*	
Teacher facilitates student responding		
Ensures that student is paying attention before providing a cue	1 2 3 4 5	
Provides clear and developmentally appropriate cues	1 2 3 4 5	
Provides cues that require responding to multiple elements (multiple cues)	1 2 3 4 5 N/A	
Summary	*1 2 3 4 5*	
Teacher provides appropriate consequences		
Presents consequence immediately, based on student's response	1 2 3 4 5	
Presents reinforcement that is naturally related to the activity or behavior	1 2 3 4 5	
Rewards good trying to encourage student to try again	1 2 3 4 5	
Summary	*1 2 3 4 5*	
Teacher prepares for session and manages environment		
Identifies effective reinforcing and motivating materials	1 2 3 4 5	
Eliminates distractions from the teaching environment	1 2 3 4 5	
Maintains control of instructional materials	1 2 3 4 5	
Uses prompts effectively	1 2 3 4 5	
Adjusts affect appropriately to match student's needs	1 2 3 4 5	
Summary	*1 2 3 4 5*	

CPRT Feedback

Date: _____   Teacher: _____

Observer: _____

Summary of observation:

1. What went well during the time you observed?

2. What elements of CPRT were used correctly? Give examples from the session.

3. What elements of CPRT were not used correctly? Give examples from the session.

4. How can the teacher improve his/her use of specific elements of CPRT?

5. Does the teacher have any questions? Please document.

6. What was the best aspect of the session you observed?

Classroom Weekly Memo

Dates: _____

Classroom News:

Student Updates:

Student	New Maintenance	New Acquisition	Preferences/Other

CPRT in the Classroom

Dear Parents,

One intervention we use in our classroom is called Classroom Pivotal Response Training, or CPRT. This handout briefly describes CPRT, so that you can be familiar with one way we are addressing your child's communication, play, social, and academic goals. Because CPRT is a naturalistic intervention, it requires no special setting, materials, or set-up. In fact, when CPRT is being implemented, it may be difficult to see the components. It can look just like play, or simply seem like "good teaching." Don't be fooled! CPRT has specific, evidence-based components, which are based on the principles of Applied Behavior Analysis (ABA). The structure and components of CPRT are described below.

ABC: CPRT is implemented in an Antecedent–Behavior–Consequence (ABC) pattern, similar to other ABA-based interventions. Children with autism often need support to learn from the natural environment. Specifically setting up opportunities to learn and providing rewards for positive behaviors give CPRT interactions structure and help children understand what to do. They can then better learn to use these new skills in many different environments. The diagram below describes the pattern and gives an example:

ANTECEDENT	BEHAVIOR	CONSEQUENCE
SEES A TOY ON A SHELF	POINTS TO THE TOY	IS HANDED THE TOY
What happens before	How the child responds	What happens after

Consequences control how likely your child is to use the same behavior in the future. If a behavior is followed by a desired consequence (receiving a favorite toy), your child is likely to use that behavior again. If a behavior is followed by an undesired consequence (being ignored), your child is likely to use that behavior less in the future.

Components: The boxes below show the structure of CPRT and list the specific components:

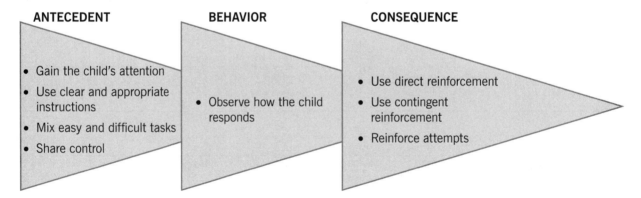

ANTECEDENT
- Gain the child's attention
- Use clear and appropriate instructions
- Mix easy and difficult tasks
- Share control

BEHAVIOR
- Observe how the child responds

CONSEQUENCE
- Use direct reinforcement
- Use contingent reinforcement
- Reinforce attempts

Tracking Progress: Data are collected regularly throughout CPRT implementation to track progress and plan instruction. Data collection is flexible, and information can be gathered at several levels of detail during both individual and group interactions.

If you'd like more information about CPRT, including a description of the components and activity suggestions for implementing CPRT at home, just ask!

CPRT en la Clase

Estimados Padres,

Una intervención que utilizamos en la clase se llama Entrenamiento de Respuesta Fundamental, o "CPRT." Esta hoja informativa describe brevemente lo que es CPRT, para que usted pueda aprender una manera en cual nosotros estamos dirigiendo las metas de comunicación, juego, sociales, y académicas de su hijo. Debido a que CPRT es una intervención naturalista, no require de materiales o entornos o posiciones especiales. De hecho, cuando se utiliza CPRT, puede ser difícil identificar los elementos. Puede verse como un juego o simplemente parecer una "buena enseñanza" con su hijo. ¡No se deje engañar! Hay elementos específicos, basado en la evidencia, que forman parte de CPRT y son basados en los principios de Análisis de Comportamiento Aplicado (ABA). La estructura y los elementos de CPRT son descritos abajo.

ABC: CPRT es implementado por parte del modelo Antecedente–Comportamiento–Consecuencia (ABC), que es similar a otros intervenciones que son basadas en ABA. Niños con autismo a menudo necesitan apoyo para aprender de su medio ambiente. Configurando oportunidades para aprender y proporcionando recompensas para comportamientos positivos hace que haya estructura en las interacciones de CPRT y ayuda al niño entender lo que tiene que hacer. Entonces pueden aprender de una mejor manera como utilizar estas nuevas habilidades en diferentes ambientes. El diagrama abajo describe el patrón y da un ejemplo:

ANTECEDENTE	COMPORTAMIENTO	CONSECUENCIA
VE UN JUGETE EN EL ESTANTE	SEÑALA CON EL DEDO AL JUGETE	CONSIGUE EL JUGET
Lo que pasa primero	*Como reacciona el niño*	*Lo que pasa despues del comportamiento*

Consecuencias controlan que tan probablemente su hijo va usar el mismo comportamiento en el futuro. Si una consecuencia positiva (recibiendo un juguete preferido) sigue un comportamiento, es más probable que su hijo va repetir ese comportamiento. Si al comportamiento le sigue una consecuencia no deseada (ser ignorado), lo más probable es que su hijo no se comporte de esa manera en el futuro.

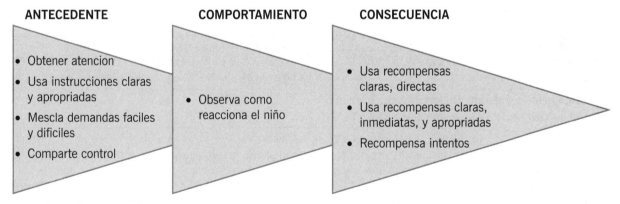

Anotando Progreso: Datos son recopilados regularmente durante la aplicación de CPRT para anotar el progreso y para planear instrucción. Colección de datos es flexible, y información puede ser recopilada en varios niveles de detalles durante interacciones individuales y de grupo.

Si quiere más información sobre CPRT, incluyendo una descripción de los componentes y sugerencias de actividades para la aplicación de CPRT en el hogar, por favor pregunte.

CPRT at Home

Thank you for your interest in CPRT! This handout is designed to describe the components of CPRT and provide examples of how to implement CPRT at home. When you use CPRT at home, learning can occur in your child's natural environment and in a wider variety of activities and settings. Using strategies consistent with how your child learns at school will help your child learn new skills faster, use skills more consistently, and better maintain skills over time. CPRT utilizes naturally occurring opportunities centered on your child's motivation to teach new skills. Since you know your child best, you are well on your way to being a CPRT expert!

> The basic structure of CPRT follows an Antecedent–Behavior–Consequence pattern:
>
> 1. **A**ntecedent: You present your child with an opportunity to respond.
> 2. **B**ehavior: Your child acts in response to that opportunity.
> 3. **C**onsequence: You provide a response to your child's behavior.

CPRT PROCEDURE

CPRT can be used within many daily activities and routines that you already do with your child! The first step is to identify motivating activities and materials. For example, if your child is particularly motivated to play a computer game, you can teach skills around asking to play this game, commenting on the events of the game, or taking turns on the computer with siblings. CPRT may be less appropriate for times when your child cannot be motivated by any aspect of the activity, as sometimes happens with self-help skills like toothbrushing or toilet training.

CPRT starts with presenting a cue for your child to respond. There are many types of cues you can use to indicate you are expecting a response. It is important to vary the type of cue you use, so that your child will learn to respond to the variety of cues presented naturally in the environment. The table below lists several different types of cues you may use in CPRT:

LANGUAGE CUES	OTHER CUES
Verbal model—Model exactly what you want your child to say ("Ball"), or start a known phrase for your child to finish ("Ready, set ... ").	Gesture or play action—Model the action you want your child to complete (roll a car or point to an item out of reach).
Instruction—Make a clear, direct statement of what you want your child to do ("Put your shoes on" or "Sit down").	Facial expression—Give an expectant look while you wait for a response (raise your eyebrows while holding a snack).
Question—Ask a brief question, either between two choices ("Red or yellow?") or open-ended ("Which movie?").	Situational—Naturally block or control access to reinforcing items (fill a drink only a little, or put a toy on a high shelf).
Comment—Make a leading statement to draw attention toward something ("Your shoes are in the kitchen").	

No matter what type of cue you use, each opportunity to respond should follow the specific components of CPRT. The components of CPRT can be broken down into antecedent and consequence components. Antecedent components occur when you present an opportunity to respond. Consequence components occur when you respond to your child's behavior. All these strategies are designed to maximize your child's motivation to participate in the interaction and minimize frustration while learning new skills.

(cont.)

ANTECEDENT ⟶ BEHAVIOR ⟷ CONSEQUENCE

ANTECEDENT STRATEGIES

1. ATTENTION—Before presenting an instruction or cue, get your child's attention. You can gain attention by controlling access to favorite items, being animated, or joining your child's play.

2. CLEAR AND APPROPRIATE INSTRUCTION—Provide instructions that are at or slightly above your child's current level of communication. Speak slowly and use direct language to improve responding.

3. EASY AND DIFFICULT TASKS—Mix in easy, already mastered tasks (maintenance) with newer, difficult skills (acquisition) to promote continued use of learned skills and keep your child's feelings of success high while learning.

4. SHARED CONTROL—Allow your child to choose materials or the activity (as long as it is not dangerous). Follow your child's interest to ensure that your child is motivated to respond. Also, take your own turns within the activity to model new actions, as well as gain access to the materials.

CHILD'S RESPONSE

CONSEQUENCE STRATEGIES

1. DIRECT REWARDS—Provide natural rewards to your child that relate to the activity. That is, reward with the preferred item or activity you and your child are talking about or playing with.

2. CONTINGENT CONSEQUENCES—Respond to your child based on their behavior. If your child responds positively, follow with a desired consequence. However, if your child does not respond positively, withhold the positive consequence and have the child try again.

3. REWARD ATTEMPTS—Reward your child for a good try, even if the behavior isn't perfect or the best your child can do. Following good attempts with desired consequences makes trying more likely in the future.

Responding to Your Child

Once you present an opportunity to respond and observe your child's response, you must react to that response by providing a consequence. CPRT uses direct, naturally occurring rewards, such as receiving a requested item or being allowed to continue with a favorite activity. The consequences you provide to your child's response determines how likely that response is to occur in the future. Behaviors followed by desired consequences will occur more often in the future, while behaviors followed by undesired consequences will decrease in the future.

As you can see, the basics of CPRT are probably not very different from the way you already interact with your child. Things that may be different, however, are being deliberate about providing opportunities to respond with clear expectations, and presenting direct consequences based on your child's behavior.

ACTIVITY SUGGESTIONS FOR HOME

You can incorporate CPRT in many activities that you already do with your child. Below are some suggested activities to get you started generating ideas, but this list is far from complete. CPRT can be used in any activity where your child is motivated by some aspect (even if it is flushing the toilet!). Be creative and have fun!

Snack Time

- Serve your child's favorite snacks and drinks in small portions, requiring him/her to request the snack items several times. Repeated practice helps support skill growth!

- Give your child snacks still in the packaging. This will require him/her to initiate and communicate with you to get the snack open.

- Serve favorite snacks without the necessary utensils (such as ice cream without a spoon) to help your child make requests.

- Be silly in the way you serve meals or snacks, so your child has to tell you each step of the process. For example, put a jar of peanut butter on a piece of bread and give it to your child!

(cont.)

Play Time

- Keep favorite toys on a high shelf or in clear plastic containers where your child can see them but not access them without your help.
- Watch a video with your child for a few minutes. Occasionally pause the video to give your child an opportunity to request that the video continue to play.
- Take a turn playing your child's favorite computer game. Do the wrong thing in the game and have your child communicate to correct you.
- Join your child while he/she is playing with a favorite toy. Model a new action with the toy and help the child complete that action, and then join in playing his/her way as a reward.

Bath Time

- Find fun water toys that require winding to operate. Your child will probably need your help to activate the toy repeatedly.
- If possible, use bath crayons to draw on the walls. You can take turns drawing with your child, have your child request items for you to draw, or draw things for your child to label.

Folding Laundry

- Your child may enjoy being covered in a warm pile of laundry. Have your child help you carry laundry from the dryer, and then bury him/her in the clothes as a reward.

Homework

- Provide your child choices during homework time, such as where to complete homework, in what order to do the problems, or what writing utensil to use. Mix easy problems with more difficult ones to keep motivation high, and reward a good try on a difficult section. You can also take turns by completing a few of the problems or sections yourself.

MORE INFORMATION

- *www.autismspeaks.org/video/glossary.php*
- *education.ucsb.edu/autism*
- Koegel, Robert L., & Koegel, Lynn Kern. (2006). *Pivotal Response Treatments for Autism: Communication, Social, and Academic Development.* Baltimore: Paul H. Brookes.

CPRT en el Hogar

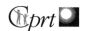

¡Gracias por su interés en CPRT! Esta hoja informativa describe los componentes de CPRT y da ejemplos para aplicar CPRT en el hogar. Cuando usted use CPRT en su hogar, su hijo puede aprender en su medio ambiente y en una amplia variedad de actividades y entornos. Usando estrategias consistentes a como su hijo aprende en la escuela ayudara a su hijo aprender nuevas habilidades más rápido. También podrá usar sus habilidades constantemente y va poder mantener sus habilidades a largo plazo. CPRT utiliza las oportunidades que naturalmente ocurren y motiva su hijo para aprender nueva habilidades. ¡Usted conoce a su hijo mejor, entonces usted va poder ser experto en CPRT!

La estructura básica de CPRT sigue el patrón de Antecedente–Comportamiento–Consecuencia:

1. **A**ntecedente: usted le presenta una oportunidad para que responda su hijo

2. **C**omportamiento: su hijo reacciona a la oportunidad para responder

3. **C**onsecuencia: usted proporciona una respuesta al comportamiento de su hijo

PROCEDIMIENTOS DE CPRT

¡CPRT se puede usar en varias actividades y rutinas diarias que usted ya hace con su hijo! El primer paso es identificar actividades y materiales que motivan a su hijo. Por ejemplo, si su hijo le gusta mucho un juego de computadora, usted puede enseñarle habilidades que pertenecen al juego. Puede enseñarle a su hijo como pedir permiso para jugar el juego, comentar sobre el juego o tomar turnos en jugar con sus hermanos. CPRT puede ser menos apropiado durante tiempos que su hijo no se pueda motivar por alguna parte de la actividad. Esto puede ocurrir en actividades tales como lavandose los dientes o durante el entrenamiento para ir al baño.

CPRT empieza con presentado una referencia para que responda su hijo. A varios tipos de referencias que usted puede usar para indicar que require una respuesta. Es importante que cambie el tipo de referencia que da para que su hijo aprenda a responder a una variedad de referencias que se presentan en su medio ambiente. El cuadro abajo da una lista de diferentes tipos de referencias que usted puede usar en CPRT:

REFERENCIAS PARA LENGUAJE	OTRAS REFERENCIAS
Modelo verbal—Modele exactamente lo que quiera que diga su hijo ("Pelota") o empiece con una frase que pueda terminar su hijo ("Una, dos … ")	Gesto o acción de—Modele la acción que quiere que haga su hijo (empuje el carro o señale con su dedo un objeto).
Instrucción—de una clara, directa instrucción que diga lo que quiere que haga su hijo ("Ponte los zapatos" o "Siéntate").	Expresión de cara—De una mirada de anticipación cuando espera una respuesta (suba las cejas a la misma vez que detenga un aperativo).
Pregunta—De una breve pregunta que sea de dos opciones ("¿Rojo o amarillo?") o general ("¿Cuál película?").	Situacional—Bloque o controle acceso a objetos preferidos (llene el vaso un poco, o pon el juguete en un estante alto).
Comentar—Haga una declaración que guie la atención a algo ("Tus zapatos están en la cocina").	

No importa qué tipo de referencia use. Cada oportunidad para responder debe seguir componentes de CPRT. Los componentes de CPRT se pueden partir en componentes de antecedentes, que ocurren cuando usted de la referencia, y componentes de consecuencias, que ocurren cuando usted reacciona al comportamiento de su hijo. Todas estas estrategias son designadas para maximizar la motivación para participar en interacciones y minimizar la frustración durante el aprendizaje de nuevas habilidades.

(cont.)

ANTECEDENTE ──────────▶ COMPORTAMIENTO ◀────────▶ CONSECUENCIAS

ESTRATEGIAS PARA ANTECEDENTES

1. ATENCIÓN—Antes de presentar una instrucción o referencia, gana la atención de su hijo. Para ganar atención, controle acceso a objetos favoritos, sea animado, o comience a jugar con su hijo.

2. INSTRUCCIONES CLARAS Y APROPIADAS— Proporcione instrucciones que sean al mismo nivel o un poco arriba del nivel de comunicación de su hijo. Hable despacio y use lenguaje directo para mejorar respuestas.

3. DEMANDAS FACILES Y DIFICILES—Mescle habilidades fáciles (mantenimiento) con nuevas, mas difíciles habilidades (adquisición). Esto va promover el uso de habilidades que ya se han aprendido y va asegurar que su hijo mantenga la sensación de éxito alta durante el aprendizaje.

4. COMPARTE CONTROL—Permita que su hijo escoja materias o actividades (que no sean peligrosas). Siga el interés de su hijo para asegurar que este motivado para responder. También tome su propio turno en las actividades para modelar nuevas acciones y ganar acceso a los materiales.

RESPUESTA DEL NINO

ESTRATEGIAS PARA CONSECUENCIAS:

1. RECOMPENSAS DIRECTAS—Proporcione recompensas naturales que son relacionadas con la actividad. Recompense con el objeto preferido o actividad que usted y su hijo estén hablando sobre o estén jugando.

2. CONSECUENCIAS CLARAS, INMEDIATAS Y APROPIADAS—Responda al comportamiento de su hijo. Si su hijo responde positivamente, siga el comportamiento con una consecuencia deseada. Si su hijo no responde positivamente, no le dé la consecuencia positiva. Haga que intente otra vez.

3. RECOMPENSA INTENTOS—Recompense a su hijo por intentos aunque el comportamiento o respuesta no sea perfecta o lo mejor que pueda hacer su hijo. Su hijo va intentar más seguido en el futuro cuando consecuencias deseadas sigan los intentos.

Respondiendo a Su Hijo

Cuando presente una oportunidad para responder y observa la respuesta de su hijo, debe de reaccionar a la respuesta con una consecuencia. CPRT usa recompensas, directas que ocurren naturalmente como recibiendo un objeto deseado o teniendo permiso para continuar con una actividad preferida. Las consecuencias que usted proporcione va determinar que tan seguido esa respuesta ocurrirá en el futuro. Comportamieentos que son seguidos con una consecuencia preferida ocurrirán más seguidos en el futuro, y a la misma vez comportamientos que son seguidos con una consecuencia que no es preferida reducirán en el futuro.

Puede ver que, los elementos básicos de CPRT no son muy diferentes de cómo usted ya interactúa con su hijo. Lo que puede ser diferente, es proporcionando oportunidades para responder con claras expectativas y presentando consecuencias directas dependiendo en el comportamiento de su hijo.

SUGERENCIAS PARA ACTIVIDADES EN EL HOGAR

Usted puede incorporar CPRT en varias actividades que ya hace con su hijo. Aquí tiene algunas actividades sugeridas para comenzar a provocar ideas. Esta lista solo tiene unas (no todas) actividades. CPRT se puede usar con cualquier actividad que motiva a su hijo en cualquier aspecto (¡aunque sea vaciando la taza del baño!). ¡Se creativo y diviértase!

(cont.)

Hora de Comida

- Sirva las comidas y bebidas preferidas en pequeñas porciones. Requiera que su hijo pida la comida/bebidas varias veces. ¡Practica repetida ayuda habilidades!

- De la comida en paquetes que no estén abiertos. Esto va requerir que su hijo inicie y comunique con usted para que abras el paquete.

- Sirva comida favorito sin utensilios (como un helado sin cuchara) para ayudar a su hijo que solicite lo que necesita.

- Has errores cuando sirvas comida para que su hijo le tenga que decir los pasos del proceso. Por ejemplo, pon la jarra de mermelada arriba del pedazo de pan y dáselo a su hijo.

Hora de Jugar

- Pon juguetes favoritos en un estante alto o en una caja de plástico claro donde su hijo pueda ver el juguete pero necesita ayuda para agarrarlo.

- Vea un video con su hijo por unos minutos. Para el video para dar una oportunidad que pida que sigan viendo el video.

- Toma turnos cuando juegan el juego favorito de su hijo en la computadora. Equivóquese a propósito durante el juego para que su hijo tenga que corregirlo.

- Cuando su hijo este jugando con su juguete favorito modela una acción nueva y ayúdelo para completar la acción y luego siga jugando como su hijo quiera para recompensar.

Hora de Bañar

- Encuentre juegos para la tina que requieren ayuda para operar. Su hijo va necesitar ayuda para jugar con el juguete.

- Si es posible, use crayolas para la tina y dibuje sobre las paredes. Puede tomar turnos dibujando con su hijo, su hijo puede pedir que dibujas algo o puede dibujar cosas que su hijo pueda identificar.

Doblando Ropa

- Su hijo puede disfrutar estar debajo ropa caliente después de salir de la secadora. Has que su hijo le ayude a cargar la ropa de la secadora y para recompensar se puede acostar en la ropa.

Tarea

- Proporciona opciones durante la hora de tarea. Por ejemplo, donde hacer la tarea, en qué orden, y que lápiz o pluma va usar. Mescla problemas fáciles con más difíciles para mantener la motivación y recompensa intentos. También puede tomar turnos en completar algunos problemas usted misma.

MÁS INFORMACIÓN

- *www.autismspeaks.org/video/glossary.php*

- *education.ucsb.edu/autism*

- Koegel, Robert L., and Koegel, Lynn Kern. (2006). *Pivotal Response Treatments for Autism: Communication, Social, and Academic Development*. Baltimore: Paul H. Brookes.

CPRT Update—
From Classroom to Home

Student: _____ Date: _____

Below are a few goals we are working on with CPRT at school:

1. Goal: _____

    Maintenance skill: _____ Acquisition skill: _____

    Home activity suggestion: _____

2. Goal: _____

    Maintenance skill: _____ Acquisition skill: _____

    Home activity suggestion: _____

3. Goal: _____

    Maintenance skill: _____ Acquisition skill: _____

    Home activity suggestion: _____

These materials and activities were especially motivating at school this month:

_____   _____

_____   _____

_____   _____

Circle the elements of CPRT that are particularly helpful:

Gaining attention   Providing clear and appropriate instructions   Using easy and difficult tasks

Sharing control   Using direct rewards   Using contingent rewards   Rewarding attempts

Notes, tips, and stories to share:

CPRT Actualización—
De la Clase al Hogar

Estudiante: _____ Fecha: _____

Metas de CPRT:

1. Meta: _____

   Habilidades para mantener: _____ Habilidades para adquirir: _____

   Sugerencia para actividades en el hogar: _____

2. Meta: _____

   Habilidades para mantener: _____ Habilidades para adquirir: _____

   Sugerencia para actividades en el hogar: _____

3. Meta: _____

   Habilidades para mantener: _____ Habilidades para adquirir: _____

   Sugerencia para actividades en el hogar: _____

Estas actividades y materiales fueron especialmente motivadoras para el estudiante este mes en la escuela:

_____   _____

_____   _____

_____   _____

Circule los elementos de CPRT que fueron particularmente útiles:

Ganando atención   Compartiendo control

Proporcionando instrucciones claras y apropiadas Utilizando recompensas directas

Utilizando habilidades fáciles y difíciles   Recompensas claras, inmediatas, y apropiadas

                                                   Recompensando intentos

Notas, consejos, y historias para compartir:

CPRT Update—
From Home to Classroom

Student: _____   Date: _____

Below are a few activities where we are using CPRT at home:

1. Activity: _____
   Goals/skills addressed: _____
   Best response: _____

2. Activity: _____
   Goals/skills addressed: _____
   Best response: _____

3. Activity: _____
   Goals/skills addressed: _____
   Best response: _____

These materials and activities were especially motivating at home this month:

_____   _____

_____   _____

_____   _____

Circle the elements of CPRT that are particularly helpful:

Gaining attention   Providing clear and appropriate instructions   Using easy and difficult tasks

Sharing control   Using direct rewards   Using contingent rewards   Rewarding attempts

Notes, tips, and stories to share:

CPRT Actualización—
Del Hogar a la Clase

Estudiante: _____   Fecha: _____

Actividades donde estamos utilizando CPRT en el hogar:

1. Actividad: _____
   Metas/habilidades: _____
   Mejor respuesta: _____

2. Actividad: _____
   Metas/habilidades: _____
   Mejor respuesta: _____

3. Actividad: _____
   Metas/habilidades: _____
   Mejor respuesta: _____

Estas actividades y materiales fueron especialmente motivadoras para el estudiante en el hogar este mes:

_____   _____

_____   _____

_____   _____

Circule los elementos de CPRT que fueron particularmente útiles:

Ganando atención   Compartiendo control

Proporcionando instrucciones claras y apropiadas   Utilizando recompensas directas

Utilizando habilidades fáciles y difíciles   Recompensas claras, inmediatas, y apropiadas

                                          Recompensando intentos

Notas, consejos, y historias para compartir:

COMPONENT 1:
Student attention

Be sure your student is paying attention to you before you ask him to do or say something. Without good attention, it will be difficult for your student to respond correctly or to learn. Students with autism may have trouble paying attention.

WHAT DOES PAYING ATTENTION LOOK LIKE?

Students with autism may be paying attention even if they are not looking right at you. Look for other signs of attention, such as a child's turning his body toward you, reaching, pointing, imitating your actions or sounds, or looking at you out of the corner of his eye. You should identify which behaviors indicate attention for individual students.

WHAT DOES NOT PAYING ATTENTION LOOK LIKE?

Sometimes it is clear that a student is not paying attention. For example, behaviors such as crying, hand flapping, repeating sounds, and walking away all indicate that your student is not attending. Other behaviors may be harder to notice. A student who is facing you but holding a toy he really likes may or may not be paying attention to you. A student who is sitting next to you at a table but staring up toward the corner may or may not be attending to you. In these situations, you should rely on what you know about the student to decide. If you have to repeat yourself several times, this is a sure sign that the student is not paying attention. Stop repeating, gain the child's attention, and then give the instruction again in a clear, simple way.

INDICATORS OF ATTENTION

- Looking toward the teacher (maybe out of the corner of the eye)
- Looking toward the teaching materials
- Body is oriented toward the teacher or materials
- Not engaged in self-stimulatory behavior
- Not playing with an object
- Reaching for teaching materials or toy

WAYS TO GAIN A STUDENT'S ATTENTION BEFORE GIVING AN INSTRUCTION

Choose motivating activities. Use toys and activities that your student enjoys. Your student may enjoy puzzles or cars and can ask for those by using sounds, words, or phrase speech. One toy can be used for many activities. A block may be used initially to teach constructive play or word imitation, and later as a "cookie" to teach symbolic play. You can add stickers your student likes to worksheets, make a math game out of toy cars, or pretend that a fan is an airplane engine.

In group situations, it can be harder to keep every student paying attention. Try letting students take turns choosing a story or song at circle time. You can give each student an object that goes along with the lesson, and have them respond to questions and play along. Other adults can redirect the students' attention back to the activity when necessary.

Be close. Being close by and providing an opportunity for face-to-face contact will help ensure that your student is able to attend to your instructions and be successful. It is less likely that your student will attend to an opportunity you provide from across the room. You may need to touch your student on the arm to gain his attention. If your student is sitting, sit with him. If your student is standing, but is very young, you may need to squat down in order to gain his attention.

Be fun. The more you enjoy yourself, the more your students will enjoy playing with you and listening to you. Be playful, silly, and animated, and watch your students' reactions to the things you do.

COMPONENT 2:
Clear and Appropriate Instruction

AN INSTRUCTION SHOULD BE:

1. **Uninterrupted.** First, make sure the student is paying attention. Afterward, wait for the student to respond to the instruction. If you are interrupted, start over.

2. **Clear and appropriate.** The instruction should be easy for the student to understand. Use clear and developmentally appropriate language. Think about the student's current level before identifying skills that will be taught. Then give an instruction that is at, or just above, the level that the student can perform on her own.

> **Clear and Appropriate Instruction:** An instruction that is easy for the student to understand and that is at, or just above, her developmental level.

Increasing Expectations: As the student begins to master new skills and understand language and social interaction, you should make your instructions more difficult. For example, you may use longer phrases, give multistep instructions, or use commenting.

Use Both Statement and Question Formats: Include both statements and questions when communicating with students. Use a natural tone of voice (not sing-song), and be sure to ask questions and model language and play in different ways, so a student doesn't get "stuck."

Developmental Progression of Skills

Skill type	Skill level	Sample instructions at developmental level	Sample instructions above developmental level
Receptive communication	Gestural	Hold up a bucket and point inside.	Say, "Roll," or "In." Gesture may be needed to assist in responding.
	Single words	Say, "Ball," paired with open-hand prompt.	Say, "Roll the ball," or "Block goes in."
	Phrase speech	Say, "Sit in the chair."	Say, "Push the green ball."
	Reciprocal communication	Say, "Time to sit at your desk."	Say, "Get the puzzle and give it to Joe."
Expressive communication	Preverbal	Hold up ball and model pointing to it.	Hold up ball and model saying, "Ball."
	Single words	Hold up ball and wait expectantly.	Hold up ball and model saying, "Throw the ball."
	Phrase speech	Hold up ball and model saying, "Roll the ball."	Hold up ball and say, "What do you want?" or "I have a ball."
	Reciprocal communication	Hold up the ball and say, "This red ball rolls fast!"	Hold up a ball and prompt, "I'm going to toss the ball in the bucket."

(cont.)

Skill type	Skill level	Sample instructions at developmental level	Sample instructions above developmental level
Play skills	Sensory–motor	Model feeling or squishing play clay.	Model stacking rings on a peg.
	Functional play	Model putting balls in tube or completing a puzzle; provide verbal instructions.	Model feeding a doll; say, "Feed the baby."
	Early pretend play (single-step actions)	Model talking on a toy phone; say, "Talk to Mommy."	Model pouring juice from an empty pitcher and say, "Baby wants juice too."
	Multiple pretend play actions	Model feeding self, doll, and peer, then driving the car to the store to get more snacks.	Provide blanket, plates, and cups and say, "Let's have a picnic!"
	Reciprocal play	Provide costumes for role playing with peers and say, "Let's play superheroes!"	Provide board games for two players that involve turn taking during free-play time.

COMPONENT 3:
Easy and Difficult Tasks

USING BOTH EASY AND DIFFICULT TASKS

When using CPRT, you should provide a mixture of both easy and difficult tasks for students with autism. Doing this helps students feel more successful and stay motivated to learn.

A **maintenance task** is a task that a student has already learned or mastered, and that he can do easily the majority of the time he is asked. An **acquisition task** is a task that a child is learning to do or something he can do sometimes, but not every time he is asked.

It is important for you to use both types of tasks. Try to mix in maintenance tasks approximately 50% of the time between acquisition tasks. However, this may be different, depending on the student. A student who is tired and frustrated may need more maintenance tasks. On the other hand, a student who is highly motivated may benefit from more acquisition tasks.

WHY DOES THIS HELP?

Increased Motivation and Spontaneity

Motivation is key in CPRT. Having your student do easy tasks that are reinforcing will help to maintain enjoyment and motivation. Mixing in skills that need to be learned will help your student make progress.

Students with autism often have a hard time doing new things on their own, or spontaneously. These students may require a lot of prompting in order to respond or initiate communication or play, but we want to see them doing things without our help. Mixing easy and difficult tasks helps to increase spontaneity, because you can wait for a student to do an easy task on her own. This gives your student a chance to spontaneously request, play, or follow simple instructions without your help. This will boost confidence and help your student use her skills in new places and over time.

TASK DESCRIPTIONS

- **Maintenance tasks:** Tasks that the student has already learned
- **Acquisition tasks:** Tasks that the student is learning. These tasks are new to the student.

COMPONENT 4:
Shared Control

WHAT IS SHARED CONTROL?

In the classroom, the teacher is usually the person in charge of the learning environment. You usually choose the materials, location, and goals for learning. In CPRT, sharing control of the learning environment and materials is another tool to increase your student's motivation. When you choose a topic or activity, you are usually more motivated and interested to learn it. For example, you may enjoy your book club discussion more when you get to choose the book. When you incorporate things that your student enjoys into a task, she will be more likely to attend and be motivated to learn. Don't forget: It is important to have control of the materials, a clear understanding of the goals, and the ultimate responsibility for the learning interaction.

HOW TO SHARE CONTROL

Follow the Student's Choice of Materials

Find materials that the student likes and that can be used in teaching the new skill. For example, if you are working on number identification and the student enjoys playing with puzzles, then use a puzzle with numbers. The key is to provide the student with an opportunity to choose at least one portion of the activity, even if you are directing the interaction.

Follow the Student's Lead

Let the student choose when to move from one activity to another. There may be times when your student is moving too quickly from one activity to another. Or the student may be spending too much time on an activity. Here are some possible solutions for these problems:

Problem	Reason	Solution
Moves between tasks too quickly	Task is too difficult or demanding.	• Increase easy tasks. • Increase reinforcement/reward.
Moves between tasks too quickly	Student has a short attention span.	• Make sure the student indicates, "All done," and asks for next activity. • Ask student to complete tasks again.
Stays at same tasks for a long period of time	Student only prefers a few toys or activities.	• Limit availability of preferred toys and activities. • Use a visual timer.
Does not choose any activity	Student has low motivation to participate.	• Be silly. Find non-toy activities. • Do a gross motor activity.

Take Turns

Taking turns is a way to interact with your student that allows you to help the student learn appropriate language and play. Turn taking allows you to regain control of teaching materials. It is important to have your student's attention. Try to take turns playfully and naturally, model at the student's level, and include peers in turn taking whenever you can. For students who do not like to take turns, keep your turns brief, or try trading toys and modeling with a duplicate toy while the student watches.

Maintain Safety and Appropriateness

Students should never be allowed to engage in dangerous (e.g., aggressive, self-injurious) or inappropriate behavior. Sometimes you can use stereotypic or self-stimulatory behavior to teach a new skill. For example, if your student loves to jump, have her count to 10 and jump 10 times. It's important for you as the teacher to decide what is appropriate and what is not.

COMPONENT 5:
Multiple Cues (Broadening Attention)

What are multiple cues? Every time you learn a new skill, it involves paying attention to multiple cues (e.g., color and shape). In fact, most learning occurs when you make associations between two or more cues. For instance, you know that communicating "good-bye" is often done by both saying the word and waving. Attending to multiple cues in the environment is essential to learning.

Although such learning is not a problem for typically developing children, students with autism often have difficulty learning when attention to simultaneous multiple cues is required.

STIMULUS OVERSELECTIVITY

The tendency to attend to only one component of a complex cue is called **stimulus overselectivity**. Students who demonstrate this attentional deficit may have trouble identifying people whose appearance has been slightly altered, such as by a haircut, or simply the removal of eyeglasses. For example, a child did not recognize her teacher after a drastic haircut from long to short hair; the student approached her teacher and asked, "What's your name?" In this case, the child had failed to recognize more permanent cues of the teacher's appearance (facial features, body type, height, etc.), which allow most of us to recognize others even when the details of their appearance change.

HOW TO HELP YOUR STUDENTS

For many children with autism, early intervention and the use of varied instructions, materials, and examples can increase appropriate attention and responding. You can help by teaching lessons in various settings, during different activities and materials. For most of your students, this type of teaching will be sufficient to provide attention to simultaneous multiple cues, because they have learned they need to do this in order to understand the lesson and respond appropriately.

For students who have continued difficulty, you can teach using **conditional discriminations**—that is, presenting opportunities to respond for which the correct response depends upon responding to multiple cues. For example, you can ask a student to get the "green pencil" from a box of colored pens, pencils, and markers.

Examples of Materials for Teaching Multiple Cues

Material type	Specific materials	Examples
Vehicles	Type and size, type and color	Small, medium, and large examples of buses, cars, and trucks in different colors
Books	Subject and size, color and size	Large and small books of different subjects, colors
Writing utensils	Type and color	Pens, pencils, crayons, and markers in different colors
Dolls/character figurines	Size and identity	Large and small dolls of several of the student's favorite characters
Animal figurines	Type and family member	Mommy and baby animals of several types
Blocks	Quantity and color, size and color, shape and color,	Various shapes of blocks in several colors, and/or sizes
Snacks	Texture and quantity, color and type	Bite-size snacks in several textures and/or colors

IMPORTANT NOTES ABOUT MULTIPLE CUES

- Typically developing children do not reliably respond to simultaneous multiple cues until approximately 36 months of age.
- These methods are not appropriate for teaching children with autism who have a developmental age of less than 36 months.

COMPONENT 6:
Direct Reinforcement

WHAT IS DIRECT REINFORCEMENT?

Giving **direct reinforcement** means that whatever the student gets as a reward for responding correctly is directly related to what she was asked to do.

Example: Teacher hold up a car and says, "What color?" Student says, "Red." Teacher gives the student the toy car.

WHAT IS INDIRECT REINFORCEMENT?

Indirect **reinforcement** is a consequence that is not related to the behavior or response of the student.

Example: Teacher holds up a car and says, "What color?" Student says, "Red." Teacher says, "Good talking!" and gives student a high five.

REINFORCEMENT TYPES

Direct reinforcement: A consequence that is directly related to the behavior. For example, if a student says, "Car," then the student is given a car.

Indirect reinforcement: A consequence that is not related to the response. For example, a teacher holds up a picture of a car and asks, "What is it?" The student responds, "Car." The teacher then says, "Good talking!" or gives the student a piece of candy.

HOW DOES DIRECT REINFORCEMENT HELP?

Direct reinforcement helps a student learn to use skills in other environments (aside from the classroom) and with other materials. This is called **generalization**. This happens when a student learns that language can change her environment. She learns that by talking, she can get what she wants. For example, if you went to a fast-food restaurant and said, "I want a hamburger," you would be disappointed to receive a cookie or hear, "Good talking!" This would not be a direct consequence related to your behavior. Behavior that is taught using direct consequences (like those found in the real world) is more likely to be generalized, and this means that your student will continue using this behavior for longer.

WHEN SHOULD I USE INDIRECT REINFORCEMENT?

Indirect reinforcement is helpful when you are teaching a student a new skill or when a direct consequence is not available. However, in these cases the student may only perform that skill in the environment in which it was taught, because the real world does not reinforce that behavior in the same way.

Direct Reinforcement: Examples

Type	Setting	Direct	Indirect
Social	You are teaching Johnny to approach a peer and ask a question. At recess, Johnny is interested in the swings. You facilitate Johnny in approaching Tom, who is playing on the swings.	You help Johnny ask Tom for a turn on the swing, and Tom gives him a turn. You push Johnny on the swing as a reward for successfully asking Tom a question.	You help Johnny ask Tom what his favorite color is. You push Johnny on the swing as a reward for successfully asking Tom a question.
Play	You are teaching Susie to engage in symbolic play. She has chosen a toy ranch set to play with, and you prompt her to pretend that a pencil is a fence.	Susie uses the pencil as a fence, and as a consequence you allow her to play with the ranch set as she pleases.	Susie uses the pencil as a fence, and as a consequence you let her choose the song for circle time.

COMPONENT 7:
Contingent Consequences

WHAT IS A CONTINGENT CONSEQUENCE?

A **contingent consequence** is presented immediately, based on the student's behavior.

Immediate: The sooner a consequence is delivered, the more effective it will be. The more delayed the consequence is after the response, the less effective it will be.

Example of an immediate consequence: Jimmy enjoys playing with markers. His teacher wants him to draw a circle to earn the marker. She says, "Draw a circle like this," and demonstrates for Jimmy. Just as Jimmy draws the circle, another student calls out for the teacher's help. She quickly gives Jimmy the markers to play with, then assists the other student.

Appropriate: Your response must depend on what the student does. For example, if a student responds correctly or gives a good try, he should receive a reward. If the student does not respond with a good try or does not respond at all, then he should not receive a reward and should try again. Your feedback should also be clear and easy for the student to understand, so that he can make the connection between the consequence and his behavior.

Example of an appropriate consequence: Jimmy asks to draw, so his teacher gets the markers. "First practice drawing a circle," she says, "then you can have the markers." Jimmy whines, "I don't wanna draw a circle," and throws his paper on the ground—so his teacher does not give him the markers.

Contingent Consequences: Examples

Type	Setting	Contingent	Noncontingent
Language	You are reading a farm story with your class during circle time. You are asking each student to make the sound of an animal in the farm story. As Nurit makes a cow sound, you notice that Paul is also attempting to say, "Mooo." This is a relatively infrequent behavior for Paul, who is usually not communicative.	Immediately upon noticing Paul's behavior, you hand him a cow figurine. You then proceed around the circle, having the students name the animals.	You continue until you have finished having all the students in the circle name the animals. Then you turn to Paul and say, "I like the way you were saying, 'Mooo,' Paul." However, now Paul is silent.
Social	During a lesson with the whole class, Marta is being disruptive by wandering around the classroom and humming loudly instead of staying in her currently assigned work station.	As soon as Marta gets up and starts to wander, you say, "Marta, please be quiet and return to your seat." You then have a paraprofessional follow Marta back to her seat to ensure that she sits down.	When you see Marta get up and hum, you say, "Marta, what are you doing now?" and continue the lesson to the class. Marta stops humming but continues wandering around the classroom.
Academic	You are teaching Joey to identify shapes by placing them in a shape sorter. Upon hearing you say, "Circle," Joey puts the circle in the correct hole.	You exclaim, "Yes, that's a circle, Joey!" and allow him to line the remaining shapes up on the floor for a few seconds before holding up the next shape for him to put in.	You then say, "Now put in the square," which Joey does successfully. Next, you hand Susie a triangle and say, "Put in." Joey loses interest and walks away from the activity.

COMPONENT 8:
Reinforcement of Attempts

WHAT IS AN ATTEMPT?

An **attempt** is a behavior that does not have the accuracy of a "correct" response but shows that the student is trying. An attempt serves the same function as the target skill or correct response.

WHY AND HOW TO REINFORCE ATTEMPTS

You should reinforce your student's attempts, even if an attempt is not her best response. This is because what may be easy for a student with autism on Monday may be hard on Tuesday, even if she is trying to do a good job. By reinforcing "good trying," you encourage more trying in the future.

Example target: "Car."

Example attempt: "Cah."

The response should be reasonably close to what you are looking for. The attempt should also be reasonably close to what the student has shown she can do in the past. Reinforcement of attempts will increase your student's motivation; she will be less frustrated, will enjoy learning more, and will be less likely to engage in difficult behaviors.

Reinforcement of Attempts: Examples

Type	Setting	Attempt reinforced	Attempt not reinforced
Turn taking	Gina and Ken are learning to share. While Ken is quite verbal and can ask for a turn, Gina is just learning. While playing with a Mr. Potato Head, Ken takes a turn and puts on the eyes. Gina picks up the mouth to put on the toy. You prompt Gina to say, "Turn," and reach for the toy. Gina has never said, "Turn," but this time she says, "Tah."	You immediately help Ken give Gina the toy and praise her for good trying.	You prompt "Turn" again, because you are working on Gina's using the whole word. Gina repeats "Tah" and reaches for Mr. Potato Head. You slowly repeat "Turn" a third time, and Gina becomes frustrated and throws the mouth at Ken.
Language	You are teaching Samir to ask for desired objects and activities by combining a verb with a noun. You see Samir reaching for a drum and prompt him to say, "Play drum." Samir says, "Pluh." You have heard Samir say the words "Play" and "Drum" very clearly many times in the past.	You wait for Samir to give a more correct response, because he is highly motivated for the drum. Samir does not, so you again prompt, "Play drum." Now Samir says, "Pluh druh," and you give him the drum as a reward for his good trying.	You give Samir the drum immediately, without waiting for a more correct response. Samir will probably not be motivated to give his best response next time. (Notice that different responses are expected for Gina and Samir, because they are at different levels.)
Play	Heather likes to play with the ring stacker, but she has trouble putting the rings on the peg. She prefers to spin the rings rather than stack them. After Heather picks up the red ring, you say, "Put red ring on." Heather starts to spin the ring, and you gently interfere with the spinning and move Heather's hand toward the peg. Heather stops spinning the ring and holds it close to the peg.	You help Heather complete the remainder of the action and put the ring on the peg while saying, "Wow, you put it on!" and allow her to spin the ring briefly as a reward for putting the ring on. Heather picks up the next ring and holds it close to the peg.	You tell her, "No, put it on the ring," and put the ring back on the floor for Heather to try again. Heather picks up the ring, starts spinning it again, and resists all further prompts.

Glossary

ABC pattern of behavior: Also called a **three-part contingency.** An **operant model** consisting of three main components: an **antecedent,** a **behavior,** and a **consequence.**

Acquisition tasks: Tasks that the student is learning. These tasks are new to the student.

Antecedent: An event or experience that happens before a behavior and is the stimulus that occasions or triggers the behavior. An antecedent can be a verbal opportunity, such as a question or instruction, or a nonverbal opportunity, such as the presence of an object in the environment.

Applied Behavior Analysis (ABA): The application of experimentally derived principles of behavior to improve socially significant actions of an individual in relation to the environment.

Attempt: A behavior that does not have the accuracy of a "correct" response but shows that the student is trying. The attempt serves the same function as the target skill or "correct" response.

Autism: A pervasive developmental disorder characterized by impaired social and communication skills and by restricted, repetitive, and stereotyped patterns of behavior.

Avoidance behavior: A behavior maintained by the removal of an undesired situation or object, such as being allowed to leave the table after a tantrum. Also called **escape behavior.**

Behavior: An individual's observable response. A behavior can be appropriate or inappropriate.

Behavioral interventions: Techniques developed by the science of **Applied Behavior Analysis (ABA).**

Classroom Pivotal Response Teaching (CPRT): A naturalistic, behavioral intervention that adapts traditional **Pivotal Response Training (PRT)** specifically for use in a classroom environment.

Communicative temptations: Intentionally setting up a situation in which a student may be motivated to communicate.

Conditional discriminations: Requiring a student to discriminate items on the basis of more than one feature (e.g., shape and color).

Consequence: Something that immediately follows a behavior and serves to increase, decrease, or maintain the occurrence, duration, latency, or intensity of the behavior in the future.

Contingent: A contingent consequence is one that is presented based on the occurrence of a specific behavior. The sooner the consequence is delivered after a response, the stronger its effects.

Cue: A signal (e.g., instruction) or a feature or element of an object or situation that is used to elicit a response.

Direct reinforcement (or reward): A consequence

that is directly related to the behavior. For example, if a student says, "Car," when motivated to play with a toy car, then access to the car is a direct reinforcer.

Escape behavior: A behavior maintained by the removal of an undesired situation or object, such as being allowed to leave the table after a tantrum. Also called **avoidance behavior**.

Expectant waiting: Using a facial expression or body posture that indicates the adult is waiting for communication from the student. No other prompts are used.

Extinction: Occurs when a behavior is no longer followed by a consequence that maintained it previously. Also called **planned ignoring**.

Extinction burst: An increase in behavior after removal of reinforcement for that behavior.

Fidelity of implementation: The degree to which an intervention is implemented as it was intended to be.

Generalization: Ability to use learned skills in different places, with different people and materials.

Indirect reinforcement: A consequence that is not related to the response. For example, a teacher holds up a picture of a car and asks, "What is it?"; the student responds, "Car." The teacher then says, "Good talking!" or gives the student a piece of candy.

Individualized Education Program (IEP): A legal document created to meet the unique educational needs of a specific student, as required by the Individuals with Disabilities Education Improvement Act of 2004.

Joint attention: Sharing an experience with someone else by looking, pointing, or gesturing to an item and referring back to the other person.

Maintenance (of skills): Ability to use learned skills continually over time.

Maintenance tasks: Tasks that the student has already learned or mastered, and can do easily the majority of the time.

Multiple cues: More than one feature or element used to identify an object, such as shape, size, color, or texture.

Negative reinforcement: The removal of an undesired situation or object following a behavior, which leads to an increase in the preceding behavior. Negative reinforcement will maintain escape or avoidance behaviors.

Operant: Having influences or producing an effect.

Operant model: A model consisting of three main components: (1) an **antecedent** event or experience that happens before a behavior; (2) a **behavior** or response by the student (or lack of behavior, in some cases); and (3) a **consequence** that serves to increase, decrease, or maintain the occurrence, duration, latency, or intensity of the behavior in the future. Also called a **three-part contingency** or **ABC pattern of behavior**.

Opportunity to respond: The initial presentation of a signal for a student to engage in a behavior, action, or reply.

Pivotal Response Training (PRT): A behavioral intervention for children with autism that maximizes learning through targeting "pivotal" skills such as motivation and the ability to respond to multiple cues.

Positive reinforcement: Presentation of a desired event or item behavior following a specific behavior. Positive reinforcement will increase the strength of the behavior that the reinforcer follows.

Preference assessment: A formal, systematic way of gathering information on student preferences. Two types of preference assessment are time-based and paired-choice.

Prompt: Support provided following a cue or opportunity to respond, to ensure a successful response to a cue.

Punishment: Presentation of an undesired event or item, which leads to a decrease in the behavior it follows.

Response cost: A form of punishment where a student's behavior results in the loss of positive reinforcement. Also called **time away**.

Stimulus overselectivity: The tendency to attend to only one component of a complex cue.

Time away: A form of punishment where a student's behavior results in the loss of positive reinforcement. Also called **response cost**.

Suggested Readings

This section of the manual is intended to provide additional information about the research used to develop CPRT and the studies behind many of the topics and principles in the manual. This is not intended to be an exhaustive list of all of the references for each topic area. We are simply providing a way for you to find more about the research in each area. Looking at these resources will lead you to many other studies and resources in each topic area.

AUTISM RATES AND INCREASES IN AUTISM

Baird G, Charman T, Cox A, Baron-Cohen, S, Swettenham J, Wheelwright S, Drew A. Current topic: Screening and surveillance for autism and pervasive developmental disorders. *Archives of Disease in Childhood*. 2001;84(6):468–475.

Fombonne E. Diagnostic assessment in a sample of autistic and developmentally impaired adolescents. *Journal of Autism and Developmental Disorders. Special Issue: Classification and Diagnosis*. 1992;22(4):563–581.

Mandell DS, Palmer R. Differences among states in the identification of autistic spectrum disorders. *Archives of Pediatrics and Adolescent Medicine*. 2005;159(3):266–269.

National Research Council. *Educating children with autism*. Washington DC: National Academy Press; 2001.

AUTISM DIAGNOSIS AND CHARACTERISTICS

American Psychiatric Association. *Diagnostic and statistical manual of mental disorders*, 4th ed., Text Revision. Washington, DC: American Psychiatric Association; 2000.

Bakeman R, and Adamson LB. Coordinating attention to people and objects in mother-infant and peer-infant interactions. *Child Development*. 1984:55(4):1278–1289.

Baron-Cohen S. Autism and symbolic play. *British Journal of Developmental Psychology*. 1987:5(2):139–148.

Bates E, Benigni L, Bretherton I, Camaioni L, and Volterra V. *The emergence of symbols: Cognition and communication in infancy*. New York: Wiley; 1979.

Cox RD, Mesibov GB. Relationship between autism and learning disabilities. In: Schopler E, Mesibov

GB, eds. *Learning and cognition in autism: Current issues in autism.* New York: Platinum Press; 1995:55–70.

Harris SL, Belchic J, Blum L, Celiberti D. Behavioral assessment of autistic disorder. In: Matson JL, ed. *Autism in children and adults: Etiology, assessment, and intervention.* Belmont: Brooks/Cole; 1994:127–146.

Kasari C, Freeman S, Paparella T, Wong C, Kwon S, Gulsrud A, et al.. Early intervention on core deficits in autism. *Clinical Neuropsychiatry: Journal of Treatment and Evaluation.* 2005:2(6):380–388.

Koegel RL, Firestone PB, Kramme KW, Dunlap G. Increasing spontaneous play by suppressing self-stimulation in autistic children. *Journal of Applied Behavior Analysis.* 1974;7(4):521–528.

Lord C, Bailey A. Autism spectrum disorder. In: Rutter M, Taylor E, eds. *Child and adolescent psychiatry.* Oxford, UK: Blackwell; 2002.

Loveland K, and Landry SH. Joint attention and language in autism and developmental language delay. *Journal of Autism and Developmental Disorders.* 1986:16(3):335–349.

Rimland B. *Infantile autism: The syndrome and its implications for a neural theory of behavior.* New York: Appleton-Century-Crofts; 1964.

Schreibman, L. *Autism.* Newbury Park, CA: Sage; 1988.

Willemsen-Swinkels SH, Buitelaar JK. The autism spectrum: Subgroups, boundaries, and treatment. *Psychiatric Clinics of North America.* 2002;25(4):811–836.

Wing L. Autistic spectrum disorders. *British Medical Journal.* 1996;312(7027):327–328.

INTERVENTIONS FOR AUTISM MENTIONED IN THE MANUAL

General Applied Behavior Analysis

Alberto PA, Troutman AC. *Applied behavior analysis for teachers,* 8th ed. Upper Saddle River, NJ: Merrill/Pearson; 2009.

Baer DM, Wolf MM, Risley TR. Some current dimensions of applied behavior analysis. *Journal of Applied Behavior Analysis.* 1968;1(1):91–97.

Kearney AJ. *Understanding applied behavior analysis.* Philadelphia: Jessica Kingsley; 2008.

Discrete Trial Teaching

Lovaas OI. Behavioral treatment and normal educational and intellectual functioning in young autis-

tic children. *Journal of Consulting and Clinical Psychology.* 1987:55:1–7.

McEachin JJ, Smith T, Lovaas OI. Long-term outcome for children with autism who received early intensive behavioral treatment. *American Journal of Mental Retardation.* 1993;97(4):359–391.

Naturalistic Behavioral Interventions

Alpert CL, Kaiser AP. Training parents as milieu language teachers. *Journal of Early Intervention.* 1992;16(1):31–52.

Bondy AS, Frost LA. The Picture Exchange Communication System. *Focus on Autistic Behavior.* 1994;9(3):1–19.

Delprato DJ. Comparisons of discrete-trial and normalized behavioral intervention for young children with autism. *Journal of Autism and Developmental Disorders.* 2001;31(3):315–325.

Halle JW, Marshall AM, Spradlin JE. Time delay: A techniques to increase language use and facilitate generalization in retarded children. *Journal of Applied Behavior Analysis.* 1979;12(3):431–439.

Hancock TB, Kaiser A. The effects of trainer-implemented enhanced milieu teaching on the social communication of children with autism. *Topics in Early Childhood Special Education.* 2002;22(1):39–54.

Hart BM, Risley TR. Establishing use of descriptive adjectives in the spontaneous speech of disadvantaged preschool children. *Journal of Applied Behavior Analysis.* 1968;1(2):109–120.

Kaiser AP, Yoder PJ, Keetz A. Evaluating milieu teaching. In: Warren SF, Reichle JE, eds. *Causes and effects in communication and language intervention (Communication and language intervention series,* Vol. 1). Baltimore: Paul H. Brookes; 1992.

McGee GG, Krantz PJ, Mason D, McClannahan LE. A modified incidental-teaching procedure for autistic youth: Acquisition and generalization of receptive object labels. *Journal of Applied Behavior Analysis.* 1983;16(3):329–338.

Rogers-Warren A, Warren SF. Mands for verbalization: Facilitating the display of newly trained language in children. *Behavior Modification.* 1980;4(3):361–382.

Schreibman L. *Autism.* Newbury Park, CA: Sage; 1988.

Schreibman L, Kaneko WM, Koegel RL. Positive affect of parents of autistic children: A comparison across two teaching techniques. *Behavior Therapy.* 1991;22(4):479–490.

Schreibman L, Koegel RL. Fostering self-management: Parent-delivered pivotal response training for children with autistic disorder. In: Hibbs ED, Jensen PS, eds. *Psychosocial treatments for child and adolescent disorders: Empirically based strategies for clinical practice.* Washington, DC: American Psychological Association; 1996:525–552.

Other Interventions

Arick JR, Young HE, Falco RA, Loos, LM, Krug DA, Gense MH, et al. Designing an outcome study to monitor the progress of students with autism spectrum disorders. *Focus on Autism and Other Developmental Disabilities.* 2003:18(2):75–87.

Baranek GT. Efficacy of sensory and motor interventions for children with autism. *Journal of Autism and Developmental Disorders.* 2002:32(5):397–422.

Creedon MP, ed. *Appropriate behavior through communication: A new program in simultaneous language for nonverbal children.* 2nd ed. Chicago: Michael Reese Medical Center, Dysfunctioning Child Center Publication; 1975.

Schopler E, and Mesibov GB, eds. *Learning and cognition in autism.* New York: Plenum Press; 1995.

PRT RESEARCH PROVIDING THE BASIS FOR CPRT

General

Koegel LK, Carter CM, Koegel RL. Teaching children with autism self-initiations as a pivotal response. *Topics in Language Disorders.* 2003;23(2):134–145.

Koegel LK, Koegel RL, Harrower JK, Carter CM. Pivotal response intervention I: Overview of approach. *Journal of the Association for Persons with Severe Handicaps.* 1999;24(3):174–185.

Koegel RL, O'Dell MC, Koegel LK. A natural language teaching paradigm for nonverbal autistic children. *Journal of Autism and Developmental Disorders.* 1987;17(2):187–200.

Koegel RL, Schreibman L, Good A, Cerniglia L, Murphy C, Koegel LK, eds. *How to teach pivotal behaviors to children with autism: A training manual.* Santa Barbara; University of California, Santa Barbara, Department of Speech and Hearing Sciences; 1989.

Stahmer AC. The basic structure of community early intervention programs for children with autism: Provider descriptions. *Journal of Autism and Developmental Disorders.* 2007;37(7):1344–1354.

Stahmer AC, and Ingersoll B. Inclusive programming for toddlers with autism spectrum disorders: Outcomes from the Children's Toddler School. *Journal of Positive Behavior Interventions.* 2004;6(2):67–82.

Communication Skills

Koegel LK, Camarata SM, Valdez-Menchaca M, Koegel RL. Setting generalization of question-asking by children with autism. *American Journal on Mental Retardation.* 1998;102(4):346–357.

Koegel LK, Carter CM, Koegel RL. Teaching children with autism self-initiations as a pivotal response. *Topics in Language Disorders.* 2003;23(2):134–145.

Koegel RL, Camarata, S, Koegel LK, Ben-Tall, A, and Smith, AE. Increasing speech intelligibility in children with autism. *Journal of Autism and Developmental Disorders.* 1998;28(3):241–251.

Koegel RL, Koegel LK, and Surratt A. Language intervention and disruptive behavior in preschool children with autism. *Journal of Autism and Developmental Disorders.* 1992;22(2):141–153.

Laski KE, Charlop MH, Schreibman L. Training parents to use the natural language paradigm to increase their autistic children's speech. *Journal of Applied Behavior Analysis.* 1988;21(4):391–400.

Sze K, Koegel RL, Brookman L, Koegel LK. Rapid acquisition of speech in nonverbal children with autism: Developing typical, social, and communicative interactions in children with autism using pivotal response training and self-management. Paper presented at the annual convention of the Association for Behavior Analysis. San Francisco, CA; 2003.

Play Skills

Humphries TL. Educators' ability to teach play skills to children with autism through the use of pivotal response training. Paper presented at the annual meeting of the Florida Association for Behavior Analysis, Daytona Beach, FL; 1998.

Stahmer AC. Teaching symbolic play skills to children with autism using pivotal response training. *Journal of Autism and Developmental Disorders.* 1995;25(2):123–141.

Thorp DM, Stahmer AC, Schreibman L. Effects of sociodramatic play training on children with autism. *Journal of Autism and Developmental Disorders.* 1995;25(3):265–282.

Social Interaction

Kuhn LR, Bodkin AE, Devlin SD, Doggett RA. Using pivotal response training with peers in special education to facilitate play in two children with autism. *Education and Training in Developmental Disabilities.* 2008;43(1):37–45.

Pierce K, Schreibman L. Increasing complex social behaviors in children with autism: Effects of peer-implemented pivotal response training. *Journal of Applied Behavior Analysis.* 1995;28(3):285–295.

Pierce K, Schreibman L. Multiple peer use of pivotal response training to increase social behaviors of classmates with autism: Results from trained and untrained peers. *Journal of Applied Behavior Analysis.* 1997;30(1):157–160.

Initiations

Koegel LK, Carter CM, Koegel RL. Teaching children with autism self-initiations as a pivotal response. *Topics in Language Disorders.* 2003;23(2):134–145.

Joint Attention

Jones EA, Carr EG, Feeley KM. Multiple effects of joint attention intervention for children with autism. *Behavior Modification.* 2006;30(6):782–834.

Rocha ML, Schreibman L, Stahmer A. Effectiveness of training parents to teach joint attention in children with autism. *Journal of Early Intervention.* 2007;29(2):154–172.

Whalen C, Schreibman L. Joint attention training for children with autism using behavior modification procedures. *Journal of Childhood Psychology and Psychiatry.* 2003;44(3):456–468.

Homework

Koegel RL, Tran QH, Mossman A, Koegel LK. Incorporating motivational procedures to improve homework performance. In: Koegel RL, Koegel LK, eds. *Pivotal response treatments for autism.* Baltimore: Paul H. Brookes; 2006.

Increasing Generalization and Maintenance

Humphries TL. Effectiveness of pivotal response training as a behavioral intervention for young children with autism spectrum disorders. *Bridges: Practice-Based Research Syntheses.* 2003;2(4):1–9.

Schreibman L, Kaneko WM, Koegel RL. Positive affect of parents of autistic children: A comparison across two teaching techniques. *Behavior Therapy.* 1991;22(4):479–490.

Independent Reviews of Use of PRT

Cowan RJ, Allen, KD. Using naturalistic procedures to enhance learning in individuals with autism: a focus on generalized teaching within the school setting. *Psychology in the Schools.* 2007;44(7):701–715.

Delprato DJ. Comparisons of discrete-trial and normalized behavioral intervention for young children with autism. *Journal of Autism and Developmental Disorders.* 2001;31(3):315–325.

Humphries TL. Effectiveness of pivotal response training as a behavioal intervention for young children with autism spectrum disorders. *Bridges: Practice-Based Research Syntheses.* 2003;2(4):1–9.

Kuhn LR, Bodkin AE, Devlin SD, Doggett RA. Using pivotal response training with peers in special education to facilitate play in two children with autism. *Education and Training in Developmental Disabilities.* 2008;43(1):37–45.

Jones EA, Carr EG, Feeley KM. Multiple effects of joint attention intervention for children with autism. *Behavior Modification.* 2006;30(6):782–834.

National Autism Center. *National standards report.* Randolph, MA: National Autism Center; 2009. See also *www.nationalautismcenter.org/affiliates*

RESEARCH SUPPORTING COMPONENTS OF CPRT

Gaining Attention Naturally

Leaf RB, McEachin JJ. *A work in progress: Behavior management strategies and a curriculum for intensive behavioral treatment of autism.* New York: DRL Books; 1999.

McClannahan LE, Krantz PJ. In search of solutions to promote dependence: Teaching children with autism to use photographic activity schedules. In: Baer DM, Pinkston EM, eds. *Environment and behavior.* Boulder, CO: Westview Press; 1997:271–278.

Siegel B. *Helping children with autism learn: A guide to treatment approaches for parents and professionals.* New York: Oxford University Press; 2003.

Following Your Student's Lead/Choice

Bambara LM, Koger F, Katzer T, Davenport TA. Embedding choice in the context of daily routines: An experimental case study. *Journal of the Association for Persons with Severe Handicaps.* 1995;20:185–195.

Cole CL, Davenport TA, Bambara LM, Ager CL. Effects of choice and task preference on the work performance of students with behavior problems. *Behavioral Disorders.* 1997;22:65–74.

Kern L, Dunlap G. Curricular modifications to promote desirable classroom behavior. In: Luiselli JK, Cameron MJ, eds. *Antecedent control: Innovative approaches to behavioral support.* Baltimore: Paul H. Brookes; 1998:289–307.

Koegel RL, Dyer K, Bell LK. The influence of child-preferred activities on autistic children's social behavior. *Journal of Applied Behavior Analysis.* 1987;20(3):243–252.

Leaf RB, McEachin JJ. *A work in progress: Behavior management strategies and a curriculum for intensive behavioral treatment of autism.* New York: DRL Books; 1999.

Moes DR. Integrating choice-making opportunities within teacher-assigned academic tasks to facilitate the performance of children with autism. *Journal of the Association for Persons with Severe Handicaps.* 1998;23(4):319–328.

Wacker DP, Berg WK, Asmus JM, Harding JW, Cooper LJ. Experimental analysis of antecedent influences on challenging behaviors. In: Luiselli JK, Cameron MJ, eds. *Antecedent control: Innovative approaches to behavioral support.* Baltimore: Paul H. Brookes; 1998:67–86.

Observational Learning (Student Imitation)

Ingersoll B, Dvortcsak A. Including parent training in the early childhood special education curriculum for children with autism spectrum disorders. *Journal of Positive Behavior Interventions.* 2006;8(2):79–87.

Ingersoll B, Dvortcsak A, Whalen C, Sikora D. The effects of a developmental, social-pragmatice language intervention on rate of expressive language production in young children with autistic spectrum disorders. *Focus on Autism and Other Developmental Disabilities.* 2005;20(4):213–222.

Reinforcing Attempts

Koegel RL, Egel AL. Motivating autistic children. *Journal of Abnormal Psychology.* 1979;88(4):418–426.

Koegel RL, O'Dell M, Dunlap G. Producing speech use in nonverbal autistic children by reinforcing attempts. *Journal of Autism and Developmental Disorders.* 1988;18(4):525–538.

Using Varied Materials and Multiple Examples

Dunlap G. The influence of task variation and maintenance tasks on the learning and affect of autistic children. *Journal of Experimental Child Psychology.* 1984;37(1):41–64.

Dunlap G, Koegel RL. Motivating autistic children through stimulus variation. *Journal of Applied Behavior Analysis.* 1980;13(4):619–627.

Responding to Multiple Cues (including stimulus overselectivity and conditional discrimination)

Koegel RL, Wilhelm H. Selective responding to the components of multiple visual cues by autistic children. *Journal of Experimental Child Psychology.* 1973;15(3):442–453.

Lovaas OI, Schreibman L. Stimulus overselectivity of autistic children in a two stimulus situation. *Behaviour Research and Therapy.* 1971;9(4):305–310.

Schover LR, Newsom CD. Overselectivity, developmental level, and overtraining in autistic and normal children. *Journal of Abnormal Child Psychology.* 1976;4(3):289–298.

Using Easy (Maintenance) and Difficult (Acquisition) Tasks

Dunlap G. The influence of task variation and maintenance tasks on the learning and affect of autistic children. *Journal of Experimental Child Psychology.* 1984;37(1):41–64.

Koegel LK, Koegel RL. The effects of interspersed maintenance tasks on academic performance in a severe childhood stroke victim. *Journal of Applied Behavior Analysis.* 1986;19(4):425–430.

Neef NA, Iwata BA, Page TJ. The effects of interspersal training versus high-density reinforcement on spelling acquisition and retention. *Journal of Applied Behavior Analysis.* 1980;13(1):153–158.

Direct Response–Reinforcer Relationships

Koegel RL, Williams JA. Direct versus indirect response–reinforcer relationships in teaching autistic children. *Journal of Abnormal Child Psychology.* 1980;8(4):537–547.

Williams JA, Koegel RL, Egel AL. Response–reinforcer relationships and improved learning in autistic children. *Journal of Applied Behavior Analysis.* 1981;14(1):53–60.

Self-Stimulatory or Stereotyped Behaviors as Motivating

Baker MJ. Incorporating the thematic ritualistic behaviors of children with autism into games: Increasing social play interactions with siblings. *Journal of Positive Behavior Interventions.* 2000;2(2):66–84.

Baker MJ, Koegel RL, Koegel LK. Increasing the social behavior of young children with autism using their obsessive behaviors. *Journal of the Association for Persons with Severe Handicaps.* 1998;23(4):300–308.

Charlop-Christy MH, Haymes LK. Using objects of obsession as token reinforcers for children with autism. *Journal of Autism and Developmental Disorders.* 1998;28(3):189–198.

Wolery M, Kirk K, Gast DL. Stereotypic behavior as a reinforcer: Effects and side effects. *Journal of Autism and Developmental Disorders.* 1985;15(2):149–161.

ADDITIONAL STRATEGIES

Gray C. *The new social story book.* Rev. 10th anniversary ed. Arlington, TX: Future Horizons; 2010.

Neumann L. *Video modeling: A visual teaching method for children with autism.* 2nd ed. Brandon, FL: Willerik; 2004.

Index

Page numbers followed by *f* indicate figure; *t* indicate table.

How to Use
the CPRT DVD-ROM

The DVD-ROM accompanying this manual contains two sets of CPRT training lectures; one set is designed for teachers, and a second, less detailed set is designed to help train paraprofessional staff in your classroom. These training lectures cover several topics in the manual. Additional information about how to use these materials for training support staff can be found in Chapter 7 of the manual.

In addition, electronic versions of the reproducible forms found in Part IV of the manual are available on the DVD-ROM.

The DVD-ROM is designed to work with any computer. Simply place the disk into your computer's disk drive. The program should automatically open on your computer screen using your default Internet browser. Although the program opens in your Internet browser, you do not need online access to use the DVD-ROM. If the program does not open automatically, you can click on the icon for the disk (which can be found by clicking the My Computer icon in Windows or on the icon for the disk on your desktop on a Mac). You will see an icon labeled **start.html**. Double-click on it and the program will start in your default Internet browser.

When the program opens, you will first see a copyright notice. Click **OK** once you have reviewed the notice and you will be in the program. If you are using Internet Explorer as your default browser, upon launching the application you may see a message asking if you want to run "Active X content." Answer **Yes** to run the application.

You will see a menu on the left side of the screen. The top section, labeled *Lectures*, allows you to view the CPRT training lectures. You can choose either *For Teachers* or *For Paraprofessionals*. Clicking on either of these links will provide a menu of the available lectures for each audience. You can go back and review the lectures at any time. Choose the lecture you would like to view. Click on the title of that lecture, and the presentation will open in a new window. The narrated lecture, including video examples, will play on your computer. The scroll bar at the bottom of the screen indicates how much material is left to view. You can use the scroll bar to go back and watch something again, or to fast forward to another part of the lecture. When you have finished viewing a lecture, you can close the program or choose another lecture to view.

If you would like to view or print one of the handouts, simply click on the topic area of interest listed in the *Resources* section of the menu bar. A list of handouts related to that topic will become visible in the center of the screen. Choose the handout you would like by clicking on the title of the handout. The handout will open in a new window on your computer screen in PDF format. From there you will be able to view and print the handout.